Drug Prescribing
in Anaesthesia
and Intensive Care

To my amazing parents,
for bringing up five children and
making us what we are today.

To my wife, Leonie, for being
so supportive and understanding.

HGWP

To my friends and colleagues
in the hospital, university and
the pharmaceutical industry
for their help and inspiration.

GRP

Drug Prescribing in Anaesthesia and Intensive Care

Henry G W Paw
BPharm MR PharmS MB BS FRCA
Specialist Registrar in Anaesthesia

Gilbert R Park
MD MA BSc MBChB FRCA
Director of Intensive Care
Consultant in Anaesthesia

The John Farman Intensive Care Unit
Addenbrooke's Hospital
Cambridge CB2 2QQ

© 1996

Greenwich Medical Media
507 The Linen Hall
162-168 Regent Street
London
W1R 5TB

ISBN 1 900 151 928

First Published 1996

A catalogue record for this book is available from the British Library

Distributed worldwide by
Oxford University Press

Produced and Designed by
Derek Virtue, DataNet

Printed in Great Britain by
Ashford Colour Press Limited

CONTENTS

INTRODUCTION

There are many small books about caring for the critically ill patient, so why another, especially about drugs? The reason is because we could find no single book that would fit in a pocket that gave the information we wanted in this area. There are many books about drugs, most list every conceivable complication and problem that can occur with a drug. Many of these are large and very few specialise in the use of drugs in the critically ill. What we hope we have written is a short, concise book that explains how to use drugs safely and efficiently in the critically ill, that residents, nurses and others will find of use.

Each section has a brief introduction about the use of drugs when an individual organ fails. It is followed by a description of individual drugs that might be used to treat that organ failure. The size means that we have limited ourselves only to a discussion of what we believe are the common drugs.

When discussing an individual drug we have limited ourselves to its use in the critically ill. Thus we have not for example considered every possible adverse effect, but concentrated on those the clinician is likely to encounter. These constraints mean that this pocket book should be seen as complementary, rather than replacing the standard textbooks.

We have rigorously checked the dose based on a 70 kg adult and information about every drug. however, despite careful checking errors may have crept in. We would therefore ask readers to check our information if it seems to be wrong. In addition, we would be pleased to hear from any readers with suggestion as to how this book can be improved.

HGWP
GRP

Cambridge 1996

EXPLANATION ON HOW TO USE THIS BOOK

The format of this book was chosen to make it more 'user friendly' - allowing the information to be readily available to the reader in times of need. For each drug, there is a brief introduction about the drug, followed by the following categories:

What to use ...... for

This is the indications for the drug's use in the critically ill.

What/when not to use ...... for

This includes conditions or circumstances in which the drug should not be used - the contraindications. For every drug, this includes known hypersensitivity to the particular drug or its constituents.

How to use ......

This includes the route and dosage for a 70 kg adult. It also advises on dilutions, line compatibility, and situations where dosage may have to be modified. Line compatibility lists the drugs which may be given in the same line; this is particularly important in the ICU setting as patients may be on more drugs than there are lines available. To make up a dilution, the instruction 'made **up** to 50 ml with 0.9% saline' means that the final volume is 50 ml. In contrast, the instruction 'to dilute **with** 50 ml 0.9% saline' could result in a total volume >50 ml. It is recommended that no drug should be stored for >24 hrs after reconstitution or dilution.

How not to use ......

Describes administration techniques or solutions for dilution which are not recommended.

Adverse effects

These are effects other than those desired.

Cautions

Warns of situations when the use of the drug is not contraindicated but needs to be carefully watched. This will include drug-drug interactions.

Organ failure

Highlights any specific problems that may occur when using the drug in a particular organ failure.

KEY TO COMMONLY USED ABBREVIATIONS

ACE-I	angiotensin converting enzyme inhibitor
AF	atrial fibrillation
ACT	activated clotting time
ADH	antidiuretic hormone
APTT	activated partial thromboplastin time
ARDS	acute respiratory distress syndrome
AV	atrioventricular
BP	blood pressure
CC	creatinine clearance
CMV	cytomegalovirus
CNS	central nervous system
COAD	chronic obstructive airways disease
CPR	cardiopulmonary resuscitation
CSF	cerebrospinal fluid
CVP	central venous pressure
CVVH/D	continuous veno–venous haemofiltration/dialysis
DI	diabetes insipidus
DVT	deep vein thrombosis
ECG	electrocardiogram
EMD	electromechanical dissociation
EBV	Epstein Barr virus
FBC	full blood count
FFP	fresh frozen plasma
g	gram
GFR	glomerular filtration rate
GI	gastro–intestinal
GTN	glyceryl trinitrate
HIV	human immunodeficiency virus
HOCM	hypertrophic obstructive cardiomyopathy
hr	hour
HR	heart rate
ICP	intracranial pressure
IHD	ischaemic heart disease
IM	intramuscular
INR	international normalized ratio
IOP	intraocular pressure
IPPV	intermittent positive pressure ventiliation
IV	intravenous
K⁺	potassium

3

kg	kilogram
L	litre
LFTs	liver function tests
M-6-G	morphine-6-glucuronide
MAP	mean arterial pressure
MAOI	monoamine oxidase inhibitor
μg	microgram
mg	milligram
MI	myocardial infarction
min	minute
ml	millilitre
MRSA	methicillin-resistant *S. aureus*
NG	nasogastric route
NSAIDs	nonsteroidal anti-inflammatory drugs
PaO$_2$	partial pressure of oxygen in arterial blood
PaCO$_2$	partial pressure of carbon dioxide in arterial blood
PCAS	patient controlled analgesia system
PCP	*pneumocystis carinii* pneumonia
PCWP	pulmonary capillary wedge pressure
PE	pulmonary embolism
PO	orally
PVC	polyvinyl chloride
PR	per rectum
RR	respiratory rate
s	second
SC	subcutaneously
SL	sublingual
SVR	systemic vascular resistance
SVT	supraventricular tachycardia
TFTs	thyroid function tests
TPN	total parenteral nutrition
U&Es	urea and electrolytes
VF	ventricular fibrillation
VT	ventricular tachycardia
WFI	water for injection
WPW syndrome	Wolff-Parkinson-White syndrome

BASIC CONCEPTS

ROUTES OF ADMINISTRATION

• **Intravenous**

This is the most common route employed in the critically ill. It is reliable, having no problems of absorption, avoids first pass metabolism, and has a rapid onset of action. Its disadvantages include: increased risk of serious side-effects and the possibility of phlebitis or tissue necrosis if extravasation occurs.

• **Intramuscular**

The need for frequent painful injections, the presence of a coagulopathy (that risks developing into a haematoma, which may become infected) and the lack of muscle bulk often seen in the critically ill, means that this route is seldom used in the critically ill. Furthermore, variable absorption, because of changes in cardiac output and blood flow to muscles, posture and site of injection, makes absorption unpredictable.

• **Subcutaneous**

Rarely used, except for heparin when it is used for prophylaxis against DVT. Absorption is variable and unreliable.

• **Oral**

In the critically ill this route includes nasogastric or orogastric administration. Except for sucralfate it is rarely used to give drugs in the seriously ill patient. The effect of pain and its treatment with opioids, variations in splanchnic blood flow, and changes in intestinal transit times as well as variability in hepatic function, make it an unpredictable and unreliable way of giving drugs in the acutely ill patient.

• **Buccal and sublingual**

Avoids the problem of absorption and first pass metabolism, and it has a rapid onset time. It has been used for GTN, buprenorphine and nifedipine.

• **Rectal**

Avoids the problems of absorption and is particularly useful for paracetamol and diclofenac, of which no IV form exists in the UK. Absorption may be variable and unpredictable. It depends on how much is absorbed from the rectum and how much from the anal canal. Drugs absorbed from the rectum (superior haemorrhoidal vein) are subject to hepatic metabolism; those from the anal canal enter the systemic circulation directly.

- **Tracheobronchial**

Useful for drugs acting directly on the lungs: β_2-agonists, anti-cholinergics and corticosteroids. It offers the advantage of a rapid onset of action and a lower risk of systemic side-effects.

LOADING DOSE

An initial loading dose is given to quickly increase the plasma concentration of a drug to the desired steady-state concentration. This is particularly important for drugs with long half-lives (amiodarone, digoxin). It normally takes five half-lives to reach steady-state if the usual doses are given at the recommended interval. Thus steady-state may not be reached for many days.

There are 2 points worth noting:

- For IV bolus administration, the plasma concentration of a drug after a loading dose can be considerably higher than that desired, resulting in toxicity, albeit transiently. This is important for drugs with a low therapeutic index (digoxin, theophylline). To prevent excessive drug concentrations, slow IV administration of these drugs is recommended.

- For drugs excreted by the kidneys unchanged (gentamicin, digoxin), reduction of the maintenance dose is needed to prevent accumulation. **No** reduction in the loading dose is needed.

DRUG METABOLISM

Most drugs are lipid-soluble and therefore cannot be excreted unchanged in the urine or bile. Water-soluble drugs such as the aminoglycosides and digoxin are excreted unchanged by the kidneys. The liver is the major site of drug metabolism. The main purpose of drug metabolism is to make the drug more water-soluble so that it can be excreted. Metabolism can be divided into two types. Phase 1 reactions are simple chemical reactions including oxidation, reduction, hydroxylation or acetylation. Phase 2 reactions are conjugations with glucuronide, sulphate or glycine. Many of the reactions are catalysed by groups of enzyme systems.

ENZYME SYSTEMS

These enzyme systems are capable of being induced or inhibited. Enzyme induction usually takes place over several days; induction of enzymes by a drug leads not only to an increase in its own metabolic degradation, but often also that of other drugs. This usually leads to a decrease in effect of the drug, unless the metabolite is active or toxic. Conversely inhibition of the enzyme systems will lead to an increased effect. Inhibition of enzymes is quick, usually needing only one or two doses of the drug. Examples of enzyme inducers and inhibitors are listed below.

Inducers	Inhibitors
Barbiturates	Amiodarone
Carbamazepine	Cimetidine
Ethanol (chronic)	Ciprofloxacin
Inhalational anaesthetics	Dextropropoxyphene
Griseofulvin	(co-proxamol)
Phenytoin	Ethanol (acute)
Primidone	Etomidate
Rifampicin	Erythromycin
	Fluconazole
	Ketoconazole
	Metronidazole

DRUG EXCRETION

Almost all drugs and/or their metabolites (with the exception of the inhalational anaesthetics) are eventually eliminated from the body in urine or in bile. Compounds with a low molecular weight are excreted in the urine. By contrast, compounds with a high molecular weight are eliminated in the bile. This route plays an important part in the elimination of penicillins, pancuronium and vecuronium.

DRUG TOLERANCE

Tolerance, over time, to a drug will diminish its effectiveness. Tolerance to the effects of opioids is thought to be a result of a change in the receptors. Other receptors will become less sensitive with a reduction in their number over time when stimulated with large amounts of drug or endogenous agonist, for example catecholamines. Tolerance to the organic nitrates may be the result of the reduced metabolism of these drugs to the active molecule, nitric oxide, as a result of a depletion within blood vessels of compounds containing the sulphydryl group.

DRUG INTERACTIONS

Two or more drugs given at the same time may exert their effects independently or may interact. The potential for interaction increases the greater the number of drugs employed. Most patients admitted to an intensive care unit will be on more than one drug. Drugs interactions can be grouped into three principle sub-divisions: pharmacokinetic, pharmacodynamic and pharmaceutical.

- **Pharmacokinetic** interactions are those that include transport to and from the receptor site and consist of absorption, distribution, metabolism, and excretion.

- **Pharmacodynamic** interactions occur between drugs which have similar or antagonistic pharmacological effects or side-effects. This may be due to competition at receptor sites, or occur between drugs acting on the same physiological system. They are usually predictable from a knowledge of the pharmacology of the interacting drugs.

- **Pharmaceutical** interactions are physical and chemical incompatibilities which may result in loss of potency, increase in toxicity, or other adverse effect. The solutions may become opalescent or precipitation may occur, but in many instances there is no visual indication of incompatibility. Precipitation reactions may occur as a result of pH, concentration changes, or 'salting-out' effects.

THERAPEUTIC DRUG MONITORING

The serum drug concentration should never be interpreted in isolation and the patient's clinical condition must be considered. The sample must be taken at the correct time in relation to dosage interval.

- **Phenytoin**

  Phenytoin has a low therapeutic index and a narrow target range. Although the average daily dose is 300 mg, the dose needed for a concentration in the target range varies from 100-700 mg/day.

- **Aminoglycosides**

  Gentamicin, tobramycin and netilmicin are antibiotics with a low therapeutic index. After starting treatment, measurements should be made before and after the third dose, and repeated if the dose requires adjustment, after another 2 doses. If renal function is stable and the dose correct, a further check should be made every 3 days, but more frequently in those patients whose renal function is changing rapidly. It is often necessary to adjust both the dose and the dose interval to ensure that both peak and trough concentrations remain within the target ranges. In spite of careful monitoring, the risk of toxicity increases with the duration of treatment and the concurrent use of loop diuretics.

- **Vancomycin**

  This glycopeptide antibiotic is highly ototoxic and nephrotoxic, and monitoring of plasma concentrations is essential, especially in the presence of renal impairment.

- **Theophylline**

  Individual variation in theophylline metabolism is considerable and the drug has a low therapeutic index. Concurrent treatment with cimetidine, erythromycin and certain 4-quinolones (ciprofloxacin, enoxacin, norfloxacin) can result in toxicity due to enzyme inhibition of theophylline metabolism.

- **Digoxin**

  In the management of AF, the drug response (ventricular rate) can be assessed directly. Monitoring may be indicated if renal function should deteriorate and other drugs (amiodarone and verapamil) are used concurrently. The slow absorption and distribution of the drug means that the sample should be taken at least 6 hrs after the oral dose is given. For IV administration, sampling time is not critical.

TARGET RANGE OF CONCENTRATION

Drug	Sampling time(s) after dose	Threshold for therapeutic effect	Threshold for toxic effect
Phenytoin	*Not critical	None	20 mg/L (80 µmol/L)
Gentamicin Tobramycin Netilmicin	Peak: 1 hr after bolus or at end of infusion Trough: pre-dose	Peak: 10 mg/L	Trough: 2 mg/L
Vancomycin	Peak: 1 hr after end of infusion Trough: pre-dose	Peak:30 mg/L	Trough: 10 mg/L
Theophylline	*Not critical	10 mg/L (55 µmol/L)	20 mg/L (110 µmol/L)
Digoxin	At least 6 hrs	0.8 µg/L (1 nmol/L)	Dependent on plasma electrolytes, thyroid function, PaO_2

Not critical, but standardise for comparison

The target range lies between the lowest effective concentration and the highest safe concentration. **Efficacy** is best reflected by the peak level and **safety** (toxicity) is best reflected by the trough level. The dosage may be manipulated by altering the dosage interval or the dose or both. If the pre-dose value is greater than the trough, increasing the dosage interval is appropriate. If the post-dose value is greater than the peak, dose reduction would be appropriate.

PHARMACOLOGY IN THE CRITICALLY ILL

It is important to remember that changes of function in the liver, kidneys and other organs may result in alterations in drug effect and elimination. These changes may not be constant in the critically ill patient, but may improve or worsen as the patient's condition changes. In addition, these changes will affect not only the drugs themselves but also their metabolites, many of which may be active.

Hepatic disease

Hepatic disease may alter the response to drugs in several ways.

* Impairment of liver function slows elimination of drugs resulting in prolongation of action and accumulation of the drug or its metabolites.

* With hypoproteinaemia there is decreased protein binding of some drugs. This increases the amount of free (active) drug.

* Bilirubin competes with many drugs for the binding sites on serum albumin. This also increases the amount of free drug.

* Reduced hepatic synthesis of clotting factors increases the sensitivity to warfarin.

* Hepatic encephalopathy may be precipitated by all sedative drugs, opioids, and diuretics that produce hypokalaemia.

* Fluid overload may be exacerbated by drugs that cause fluid retention, e.g. NSAIDs and corticosteroids.

* Renal function may be depressed. It follows that drugs having a major renal route of elimination may be affected in liver disease, because of the secondary development of renal impairment.

* Hepatotoxic drugs should be avoided.

Renal impairment

Impairment of renal function may result in failure to excrete a drug or its metabolites. The degree of renal impairment can be measured using creatinine clearance, which requires 24 hr urine collection. It can be estimated by calculation using serum creatinine (see Appendix A). Serum creatinine depends on age, sex and muscle mass. Elderly patients and the critically ill may have creatinine clearances below 50 ml/min but because of reduced muscle mass, increased serum creatinine may be "normal".

When the creatinine clearance is greater than 30 ml/min, it is seldom necessary to modify normal doses, except for certain antibiotics and cardiovascular drugs which are excreted unchanged by the kidneys. There is no need to decrease the initial or loading dose. Maintenance doses are adjusted by either lengthening the interval between doses or by reducing the size of individual doses or a combination of both. Therapeutic drug monitoring, when available, is an invaluable guide to therapy.

Haemofiltration or dialysis does not usually replace the normal excretory function of the kidneys. A reduction in dose may be needed.

Nephrotoxic drugs should, if possible, be avoided in renal impairment. Those incriminated include frusemide, thiazides, sulphonamides, aminoglycosides, and rifampicin.

Cardiac failure

Drug absorption may be impaired because of GI mucosal congestion. Dosages of drugs that are mainly metabolised by the liver or mainly excreted by the kidneys may need to be modified. This is because of impaired drug delivery to the liver which delays metabolism and impaired renal function leading to delayed elimination.

EMERGENCY DRUGS

CARDIOPULMONARY RESUSCITATION: THE ERC GUIDELINES 1992

- **Algorithm for VF or pulseless VT**

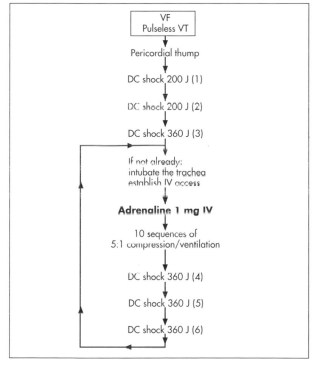

Notes:

- The interval between shocks 3 and 4 should not exceed 2 mins.
- Adrenaline should be given during each loop, i.e. every 2–3 mins.
- Consider loops for as long as defibrillation is indicated
- After 3 loops consider:
  Sodium bicarbonate 50 mmol IV
  Lignocaine 100 mg IV

DRUGS IN VF/PULSELESS VT

There is no need to delay the DC shocks for drugs. Defibrillation is still the only intervention capable of restoring a spontaneous circulation.

- **Adrenaline 1 mg (10 ml 1 in 10,000/1 ml 1 in 1,000)**

    Adrenaline has both α- and β-effects. The α-effect increases perfusion pressure and thus myocardial and cerebral blood flow. The β_1-effect helps to maintain cardiac output after spontaneous heart action has been restored and it may facilitate defibrillation by 'coarsening' the VF.

- **Sodium bicarbonate 50 mmol (50 ml 8.4%)**

    Sodium bicarbonate should be considered after every 3 loops – when acidosis may develop and perpetuate arrhythmias. Give 50 mmol of sodium bicarbonate into a central vein and recheck the plasma pH. Ideally it should be given in the knowledge of the arterial or central venous pH and bicarbonate level. Several problems are associated with its use:

    (i) CO_2 released passes across the cell membrane and causes intracellular acidosis.

    (ii) The development of an iatrogenic extracellular alkalosis may be even less favourable than acidosis.

    (iii) It may induce hyperosmolarity causing a decrease in aortic diastolic pressure and therefore a decrease in coronary perfusion pressure.

    Do not let sodium bicarbonate come into contact with catecholamines (inactivate) or calcium salts (precipitate).

- **Lignocaine 100 mg (10 ml 1%)**

    Lignocaine is no longer a first line drug in the treatment of VF. It can be of value in the prevention of VF, but there is experimental evidence that it may make defibrillation more difficult. It may be given after every 3 loops but – in the light of existing evidence – its use is not mandatory. Bretylium (5 mg/kg) and amiodarone (5 mg/kg) are alternatives.

- **Algorithm for asystole**

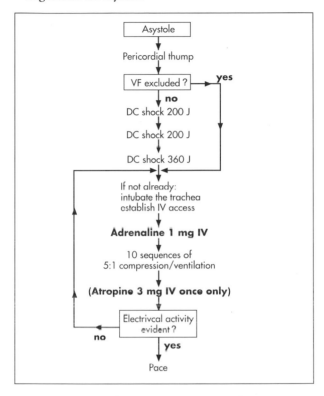

Note: If no response after 3 loops consider adrenaline 5 mg IV

DRUGS IN ASYSTOLE

- **Atropine 3 mg IV**

  This dose will block vagal tone fully, but only one dose is recommended.

- **Adrenaline**

  As in the VF algorithm, adrenaline is given to enhance basic life support. If no response has been obtained after 3 loops, high dose adrenaline (5 mg) should be considered, though its value is unproven.

- **Algorithm for EMD**

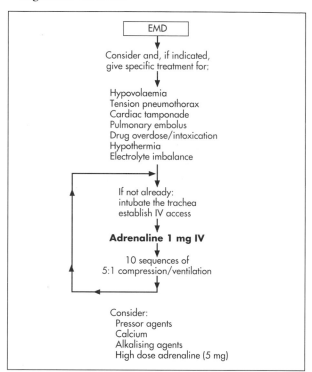

DRUGS IN EMD

The search for specific and correctable causes of EMD is of prime importance. If no evidence exists for any specific causes CPR should be continued with the use of adrenaline.

- **Calcium chloride 100 mg IV (10 ml 10%)**

Adequate levels of ionised calcium are necessary for effective cardiovascular function. Ionised calcium concentrations decrease during prolonged (>7.5 mins) cardiac arrest. The chloride salt is preferred to the gluconate salt as it does not need hepatic metabolism to release the calcium ion.

Caution: Calcium overload is thought to play an important role in ischaemic and reperfusion cell injury. Excessive doses should not be used.

Currently, there are only 3 indications for its use: hypocalcaemia, hyperkalaemia, and calcium–channel antagonist overdose.

Tracheobronchial route for drugs

If venous access is impossible, the tracheal route may be used for:

- Adrenaline
- Atropine
- Lignocaine

Drug doses are 2-3 times that of the IV route. Dilute with 0.9% saline to a total of 10 ml and instill deeply via a suction catheter or similar and give 5 big breaths. Drug absorption may be impaired by atelectasis, pulmonary oedema, and – in the case of adrenaline – local vasoconstriction.

Do not give sodium bicarbonate and calcium chloride by this route.

MANAGEMENT OF ACUTE MAJOR ANAPHYLAXIS

- **Immediate therapy**

  Stop giving the suspect drug

  Maintain airway, give 100% oxygen

  Adrenaline 50–100 µg (0.5–1 ml 1:10,000) IV
  Further 100 µg boluses as necessary for
  hypotension and bronchospasm

  Colloid 500–1000 ml rapidly

- **Secondary management**

  For adrenaline-resistant bronchospasm:
  Salbutamol 250 µg IV loading dose
  5–20 µg/min maintenance
  dilute 5 mg in 500 ml 5% glucose or 0.9% saline (10 µg/ml)
  or
  Aminophylline 5 mg/kg
  in 500 ml 0.9% saline, IV infusion over 5 hrs

  To prevent further deterioration:
  Hydrocortisone 200 mg IV
  and
  Chlorpheniramine 20 mg IV
  dilute with 10 ml 0.9% saline or WFI given over 1-2 mins

- **Investigation**
1. Take blood in an EDTA tube for plasma tryptase level at the
   following times:
   as soon as possible (within 1 hr)
   at 3 hrs
   at 24 hrs (as control)

2. Collect 10 ml urine for urinary tryptase level at the following
   times:
   as soon as possible
   at 24 hrs

MANAGEMENT OF SEVERE HYPERKALAEMIA

Criteria for treatment:
K^+ > 6.5 mmol/l
ECG changes
Severe weakness

- **Calcium chloride 10-20 ml 10% IV over 5-10 mins**
  This increases the cell depolarisation threshold and reduces myocardial irritability. It results in improvement in ECG changes within seconds, but because the K^+ levels are not altered, the effect lasts only about 30 mins.

- **Soluble insulin 15 units with 50 ml 50% glucose (50 g)**
  Given IV over 30-60 mins. Begins lowering serum K^+ in 2-5 mins and the effect lasting 1-2 hrs. Monitor blood glucose.

- **Sodium bicarbonate 50 mmol (50 ml 8.4%)**
  By correcting the acidosis its effect again is only transient. Beware in patients with fluid overload.

- **Calcium resonium 15 g PO or 30 g as retention enema, 8 hrly**
  This will draw the K^+ from the gut and remove K^+ from the body. Oral lactulose 20 ml 8 hrly may induce a mild diarrhoea which helps to remove K^+ and also avoids constipation when resins are used.

- **Haemofiltration/dialysis**
  Indicated if: plasma K^+ persistently ↑; acidosis; uraemia; or when serious fluid overload is already present.

MANAGEMENT OF MALIGNANT HYPERTHERMIA

Clinical features
Jaw spasm immediately after suxamethonium
Generalised muscle rigidity
Unexplained tachycardia, tachypnoea, sweating and cyanosis
Progressive increase in $ETCO_2$
Rapid increase in body temperature (> 4°C/hr)

Management
- Inform surgical team and send for experienced help.
  Elective surgery: abandon procedure, monitor and treat.
  Emergency surgery: finish as soon as possible, switch to 'safe agents', monitor and treat.

- Stop all inhalational anaesthetics

- Change to vapour-free anaesthetic machine and hyperventilate with **100% O_2** at 2-3 times predicted minute volume

- Give **dantrolene 1 mg/kg IV**
  Response to dantrolene should begin in minutes (decrease muscle tone, heart rate and temperature); if not, repeat every 5 mins, up to a total of 10 mg/kg.

- Give **Sodium bicarbonate 100 ml 8.4% IV**
  Further doses guided by arterial blood gas

- Correct hyperkalaemia with **50 ml 50% dextrose + 10 units insulin** over 30 mins.

- Correct cardiac arrhythmias according to their nature (usually respond to correction of acidosis, hypercarbia and hyperkalaemia).

- **Monitoring and investigations**
  ECG, BP and capnography (if not already in use)
  Oesophageal or rectal temperature: core temperature
  Urinary catheter: send urine for myoglobin and measure urine output
  Arterial line: arterial gas analysis, U & Es and creatine phosphokinase
  Central venous line: CVP and IV fluids
  Fluid balance chart: sweating loss to be accounted for

- Start **active cooling**
  Refrigerated 0.9% saline IV 1-2 litres initially (avoid Hartmann's solution because of its potassium content).
  Surface cooling: ice packs and fans (may be ineffective because of peripheral vasoconstriction).

Lavage of peritoneal and nasogastric cavities with refrigerated 0.9% saline.

- Maintain urine output with:
IV fluids
Mannitol
Frusemide

After the crisis

Admit to ICU for at least 24 hrs (crisis can recur)
Monitor potassium, creatine phosphokinase, myoglobinuria, temperature, renal failure and clotting status.
May need to repeat dantrolene (half-life only 5 hrs)
Investigate patient and family for susceptibility

Triggering agents

Suxamethonium
All potent inhalational anaesthetic agents

Safe drugs

All benzodiazepines
Thiopentone, propofol
All non-depolarising muscle relaxants
All opioids
Nitrous oxide
All local anaesthetic agents
Neostigmine, atropine, glycopyrrolate
Droperidol, metoclopramide

SEDATION, ANALGESIA AND NEUROMUSCULAR BLOCKADE

The current, ideal level of sedation should leave a patient lightly asleep but easily roused. Opioids, in combination with a benzodiazepine or propofol, are currently the most frequently used method of sedation.

The most common indication for the therapeutic use of **opioids** is to provide analgesia. They are also able to elevate mood and suppress the cough reflex. This anti-tussive effect is a useful adjunct to their analgesic effects in patients who need to tolerate a tracheal tube.

Midazolam, the shortest acting of all the **benzodiazepines** is the most widely used. It can be given either by infusion or intermittent bolus doses.

Propofol is achieving widespread popularity for sedation, although it is expensive. It is easily titrated to achieve the desired level of sedation and its effects end rapidly when the infusion is stopped, even after several days of use. Propofol is ideal for short periods of sedation on the ICU, and during weaning when longer acting agents are being eliminated. Some workers recommend propofol for long-term sedation.

At the moment all of the new sedative and analgesic drugs are designed to be short acting. This means that they usually have to be given by continuous intravenous infusion. The increased cost of these drugs can be justified if they give better control and predictable analgesia and sedation, and allow quicker weaning from ventilatory support.

NSAIDs have an opioid-sparing effect and is of particular benefit for the relief of pain from bones and joints, as well as the general aches and pains associated with prolonged immobilisation. However, their use in the critically ill is significantly limited by their side effects which include reduced platelet aggregation, gastrointestinal haemorrhage, and deterioration in renal function.

Antidepressants are useful in patients who are recovering from a prolonged period of critical illness. At this time depression and sleep disturbances are common. The beneficial effect may not be apparent until 2 weeks after starting the drug unless a large loading dose is given. Cardiovascular effects, in particular arrhythmias, have not proved to be a problem. Whether the newer quadricyclic agents will have any advantages remains to be proven.

Chlormethiazole has sedative and anticonvulsant properties It is usually reserved for patients with an alcohol problem.

Muscle relaxants are neither analgesic nor sedative agents and therefore should not be used without ensuring that the patient is both pain-free and unaware. Their use have declined since the introduction of synchronized modes of ventilation and more sophisticated electronic control mechanisms. Suxamethonium, atracurium and vecuronium are presently the most commonly used agents, although pancuronium still retains a use in ICUs. Their use should be restricted to certain specific indications:

- Tracheal intubation
- Facilitation of procedures, e.g. tracheostomy
- ARDS, where oxygenation is critical and there is risk of barotrauma
- Management of neurosurgical or head injured patients where coughing or straining on the tracheal tube increase ICP
- To stop the spasm of tetanus

Regular monitoring with a peripheral nerve stimulator is desirable; ablation of more than 3 twitches of the train-of-four is very rarely necessary.

A PRACTICAL APPROACH TO SEDATION AND ANALGESIA

The way each ICU sedates its patients will depend on many factors. The number of doctors and nurses, design of the ICU (open plan versus single rooms) and the type of equipment are but some.

Midazolam and morphine given by IV boluses (2.5 mg) is a suitable regimen if a prolonged period of ventilatory support is anticipated and the patient does not have renal or hepatic impairment. An infusion can be started if this dose is required to be given frequently. Scoring of the level of sedation is essential. Once an infusion of either drug is started then its need should be reviewed on a daily basis and its dose reduced or stopped (preferably before the morning ward round) until the patient is seen to recover from the effects of the drug. Unnecessary use of infusions may induce tolerance. It should be remembered that although analgesics may provide sedation, sedatives do not provide analgesia; agitation caused by pain should be treated with an analgesic and not by increasing the dose of the sedative.

As the patient's condition improves and weaning from ventilatory support is anticipated, the morphine and midazolam can be stopped and an infusion of propofol and/or alfentanil started. This allows any prolonged effects of midazolam and morphine to wear off.

Such a regimen is effective both in terms of patient comfort and in avoiding the use of expensive drugs.

Sedation	Analgesia	Neuromuscular Blockade
• Amitriptyline • Chlormethiazole • Flumazenil • Haloperidol • Midazolam • Propofol	• Alfentanil • Diclofenac • Fentanyl • Morphine • Naloxone • Pethidine	• Atracurium • Pancuronium • Suxamethonium • Vecuronium

AMITRIPTYLINE

A tricyclic antidepressant with sedative properties. When given at night it will help to promote sleep. It may take up to 2 weeks before any beneficial effect is seen unless a large loading dose is used.

What to use amitriptyline for
Depression in patients requiring long-term ICU stay, particularly where sedation is required.
Difficulty with sleep.

When not to use amitriptyline
Recent myocardial infarction
Arrhythmia
Heart block
Severe liver disease

How to use amitriptyline
Orally: 25-75 mg nocte
IM/IV bolus: 10-20 mg nocte

How not to use amitriptyline
During the daytime (disturbs the normal sleep pattern)

Adverse effects
Antimuscarinic effects (dry mouth, blurred vision, urinary retention)
Arrhythmias
Postural hypotension
Confusion
Hyponatraemia

Cautions
Cardiac disease (risk of arrhythmias)
Hepatic failure
Acute angle glaucoma
Concurrent use of MAOI
Additive CNS depression with other sedative agents
May potentiate direct-acting sympathomimetic drugs
Prostatic hypertrophy – urinary retention (unless patient's bladder catheterized)

Organ failure
CNS: Sedative effects increased
Hepatic: Sedative effects increased

CHLORMETHIAZOLE

Available as capsules (192 mg), syrup (250 mg/5 ml) and in a 0.8% solution for IV use. The solution contains only Na^+ 32 mmol/L and no other electrolytes. It has no analgesic effect, little cardiac and respiratory depression, and may be used in elderly patients.

Initial recovery is by redistribution, and it is eliminated by hepatic metabolism. Prolonged infusion may lead to accumulation and delayed recovery.

What to use chlormethiazole for
Sedation in the critically ill
Management of alcohol withdrawal syndrome
Anticonvulsant
Pre-eclampsia and eclampsia

When not to use chlormethiazole
As it is only available in a dilute solution for IV use, it imposes a large waterload and should be avoided if there is fluid overload or cerebral/pulmonary oedema.

How to use chlormethiazole
• For sedation
IV infusion: starting rate 25 ml/min for 1-2 mins, maintain at 1-4 ml/min
• Acute alcohol withdrawal

Orally: Day 1 9-12 capsules in 3-4 divided doses
         Day 2 6-8 capsules in 3-4 divided doses
         Day 3 4-6 capsules in 3-4 divided doses
         Then gradually reduce over days 4-6
         Do not treat for >9 days
         1 capsule $\equiv$ 5 ml syrup

IV infusion: 3-8 ml/min until sedated, but still able to obey commands. Maintain at 0.5-1 ml/min

How not to use chlormethiazole
Rapid infusion (risk of apnoea and hypotension)
Prolonged use (risk of accumulation)
Abrupt withdrawal

Adverse effects
Increased nasopharyngeal and bronchial secretions
Thrombophlebitis
Tachycardia and transient decrease in BP

Cautions

Airway obstruction in deep sedation

Cardiac and respiratory disease – confusion may indicate hypoxia

Hepatic impairment – sedation can mask hepatic coma

Renal impairment

Organ failure

CNS: Risk of cerebral oedema

Cardiac: Risk of pulmonary oedema

Hepatic: Reduced clearance with accumulation. Can precipitate coma

Renal: Increased cerebral sensitivity

FLUMAZENIL

A competitive antagonist at the benzodiazepine receptor. It has a short duration of action (20 mins).

What to use flumazenil for

To facilitate weaning from ventilation in patients sedated with benzodiazepine
In the management of benzodiazepine overdose.
As a diagnostic test for the cause of prolonged sedation.

What not to use flumazenil for

Tricyclic antidepressant and mixed-drug overdose (fits)
Patients on long-term benzodiazepine therapy (withdrawal)
Epileptic patients on benzodiazepines (fits)
Patients with increased ICP (further increase in ICP)

How to use flumazenil

Dose. 200 μg IV bolus, repeat at 1-minute intervals until desired response, up to a total dose of 2 mg.
If resedation occurs, repeat dose every 20 mins

How not to use flumazenil

Ensure the effects of neuromuscular blockade have ended before using flumazenil

Adverse effects

Dizziness
Agitation
Arrhythmias
Hypertension
Epileptic fits

Cautions

Resedation

Organ failure

Hepatic: Reduced elimination

HALOPERIDOL

A butyrophenone with longer duration of action than droperidol. It has antiemetic and neuroleptic effects with minimal cardiovascular and respiratory effects. It is a mild α−blocker and may cause hypotension in the presence of hypovolaemia.

What to use haloperidol for
Acute agitation

What not to use haloperidol for
Agitation caused by hypoxia, hypoglycaemia or a full bladder
Parkinson's disease

How to use haloperidol
IV bolus: 2.5-5 mg
IM: 5-10 mg
Up to every 4–8 hrs

How not to use haloperidol
Hypotension resulting from haloperidol should not be treated with adrenaline as a further decrease in BP may result.

Adverse effects
Extrapyramidal movements
Neuroleptic malignant syndrome (treat with dantrolene)

Cautions
Concurrent use of other CNS depressants (enhanced sedation)

Organ failure
CNS: Sedative effects increased
Hepatic: Can precipitate coma
Renal: Increase cerebral sensitivity

MIDAZOLAM

Midazolam is a water-soluble benzodiazepine with normally a short duration of action (elimination half-life 1-4 hrs). However, a prolonged coma has been reported in some critically ill patients. This has usually been after prolonged infusions. It is metabolized mostly to the metabolite 1- hydroxy midazolam which is rapidly conjugated. Accumulation of midazolam after prolonged sedation has been observed in critically ill patients. In renal failure, the glucuronide may also accumulate causing narcosis.

What to use midazolam for
Sedation
Anxiolysis

What not to use midazolam for
As an analgesic
Airway obstruction

How to use midazolam
- IV bolus: 2.5-5 mg as necessary
- IV infusion: 0.5-6 mg/hr
  Administer neat or diluted in 5% glucose or 0.9% saline
  Titrate dose to level of sedation required.
  Stop or reduce infusion each day until patient awakes, when it is restarted. Failure to assess daily will result in delayed awakening when infusion is finally stopped.
  Time to end effects after infusion: 30 mins to 2 hrs (but see below).

LINE COMPATIBILITY
- atracurium
- droperidol
- fentanyl
- metoclopramide
- morphine
- pancuronium
- vecuronium

LINE INCOMPATIBILITY
- amino acid solutions

How not to use midazolam

The use of flumazenil after prolonged use may produce confusion, toxic psychosis, convulsions, or a condition resembling delirium tremens.

Adverse effects

Residual and prolonged sedation
Respiratory depression and apnoea
Hypotension
Sexual hallucinations

Cautions

Enhanced and prolonged sedative effect results from interaction with:

- Opioid analgesics
- Antidepressants
- Antihistamines
- Alpha-blockers
- Antipsychotics

Enhanced effect in the elderly and in patients with hypovolaemia, vasoconstriction, or hypothermia.

Midazolam is metabolised by the hepatic microsomal enzyme system (cytochrome P450s). Induction of the P450 enzyme system by another drug can gradually increase the rate of metabolism of midazolam, resulting in lower plasma concentrations and a reduced effect. Conversely inhibition of the metabolism of midazolam results in a higher plasma concentration and an increased effect. Examples of enzyme inducers and inhibitors are listed on p 7.

There is now available a specific antagonist, flumazenil.

Organ failure

CNS: Sedative effects increased
Cardiac: Exaggerated hypotension
Respiratory: ↑ respiratory depression
Hepatic: Enhanced and prolonged sedative effect
            Can precipitate coma
Renal: Increased cerebral sensitivity

PROPOFOL

Propofol is an IV anaesthetic agent that has rapidly become popular as a sedative drug in the critically ill. Its major advantages are that it has a rapid onset of action and a rapid recovery even after prolonged infusion. Propofol 1% (10 mg/ml) is formulated in intralipid. A 2% formulation is available in some countries. If the patient is receiving other IV lipid concurrently, a reduction in quantity should be made to account for the amount of lipid infused as part of the propofol and avoid fat overload. One ml of propofol 1% contains 0.1 g of fat.

What to use propofol for

Sedation, especially for weaning from other sedative agents

What not to use propofol for

As an analgesic
Airway obstruction
Hypersensitivity to propofol, soybean oil, or egg lecithin (egg yolk)
Sedation in children – safety in critically ill children unknown

How to use propofol

* Sedation
  IV bolus: 10-20 mg as necessary
  IV infusion: up to 4 mg/kg/hr

Titrate to desired level of sedation - assess daily.
Measure serum triglycerides regularly.
Contains no preservatives – discard after 12 hrs.
May be diluted only with 5% glucose – mix aseptically 1 part propofol 1% with up to 4 parts 5% glucose. Stable for up to 6 hrs.

How not to use propofol

Do not give in the same line as blood or blood products

Adverse effects

Hypotension
Bradycardia
Apnoea
Pain on injection (minimised by mixing with lignocaine 1 mg for every 10 mg propofol)
Fat overload
Convulsions and myoclonic movements

Cautions

Epileptics
Lipid disorders (risk of fat overload)
Egg allergy – most patients are allergic to the egg albumin

Organ failure

CNS: Sedative effects increased
Cardiac: Exaggerated hypotension

ALFENTANIL

It is 30 times more potent than morphine and its duration is shorter than that of fentanyl. The maximum effect occurs about 1 min after IV injection. Duration of action is between 5-10 mins. Its distribution volume and lipophilicity are lower than fentanyl. It is ideal for infusion, and may be the agent of choice in renal failure. In patients with hepatic failure the elimination half-life may be markedly increased and a prolonged duration of action may be seen.

What to use alfentanil for
Patients receiving short-term ventilation

When not to use alfentanil
Airway obstruction

How to use alfentanil
- IV bolus: 500 μg every 10 mins as necessary
- IV infusion rate: 1-5 mg/hr (up to 1 μg/kg/min)

How not to use alfentanil
In combination with an opioid partial agonist e.g. buprenorphine (antagonises opioid effects).

Adverse effects
Respiratory depression and apnoea
Bradycardia
Nausea and vomiting
Delayed gastric emptying
Reduced intestinal mobility
Biliary spasm
Constipation
Urinary retention
Chest wall rigidity (may interfere with ventilation)

Cautions
Enhanced sedative and respiratory depression from interaction with:
- Benzodiazepines
- Antidepressants
- Antipsychotics

Head injury and neurosurgical patients (may exacerbate $\uparrow$ ICP as a result of $\uparrow$ $PaCO_2$)

Erythromycin ($\downarrow$ clearance of alfentanil)

Organ failure
Respiratory: $\uparrow$ respiratory depression
Hepatic: Enhanced and prolonged sedative effect

DICLOFENAC

NSAID with analgesic, anti-inflammatory, and antipyretic properties. It has an opioid-sparing effect. In the ICU, it is most conveniently given as a suppository and recently, it has been licensed for IV use.

What to use diclofenac for
Pain, especially musculoskeletal
Antipyretic

What not to use diclofenac for
Asthma (wheeze)
Hypersensitivity to aspirin and other NSAIDs (cross sensitivity)
Active peptic ulceration (bleeding)
Haemophilia and other clotting disorders (bleeding)
Renal and hepatic failure (worsening)
As a suppository in inflammatory bowel disease affecting anus, rectum and sigmoid colon (worsening of disease).

How to use diclofenac
- Pain
  PR: 100 mg suppository 18 hrly.
  IV infusion: 75 mg diluted with 50 ml 0.9% saline over 30-120 mins.
  Maximum daily dose: 150 mg.

- Antipyretic
  IV bolus: 10 mg diluted with 20 ml 0.9% saline.

How not to use diclofenac
Do not give suppository in proctitis

Adverse effects
Epigastric pain
Peptic ulcer
Rashes
Worsening of liver function tests
Prolonged bleeding time (platelet dysfunction)
Acute renal failure - in patients with:
- Pre-existing renal and hepatic impairment
- Hypovolaemia
- Renal hypoperfusion
- Sepsis

Cautions

Elderly
Hypovolaemia
Renal and hepatic impairment
Previous peptic ulceration

Organ failure

Hepatic: Diclofenac may worsen function
Renal: Diclofenac may worsen function

FENTANYL

Fentanyl is 100 times as potent as morphine. Its onset of action is within 1-2 mins after IV injection and a peak effect within 4-5 mins. Duration of action after a single bolus is 20 mins.

What to use fentanyl for

Analgesia

When not to use fentanyl

Airway obstruction

How to use fentanyl

- During anaesthesia

IV bolus: 1-3 µg/kg with spontaneous ventilation
5-10 µg/kg with IPPV
7-10 µg/kg to obtund pressor response of laryngoscopy
Up to 100 µg/kg for cardiac surgery

- For sedation

IV infusion: 1-5 µg/kg/hr

How not to use fentanyl

In combination with an opioid partial agonist e.g. buprenorphine (antagonises opioid effects).

Adverse effects

Respiratory depression and apnoea
Bradycardia and hypotension
Nausea and vomiting
Delayed gastric emptying
Reduced intestinal mobility
Biliary spasm
Constipation
Urinary retention
Chest wall rigidity (may interfere with ventilation)

Muscular rigidity and hypotension more common after high dosage

Cautions

Enhanced sedative and respiratory depression from interaction with:

- Benzodiazepines
- Antidepressants
- Antipsychotics

Head injury and neurosurgical patients (may exacerbate $\uparrow$ ICP as a result of $\uparrow$ PaCO$_2$)

Organ failure

Respiratory: $\uparrow$ respiratory depression
Hepatic: Enhanced and prolonged sedative effect.

MORPHINE

Morphine is the standard opioid to which others are compared and remains a valuable drug for the treatment of acute, severe pain. Peak effect after IV bolus is at 15 mins. Duration of action is between 2-3 hrs. Both liver and kidney function are responsible for morphine elimination. It is mainly metabolised by the liver. One of the principle metabolites, M-6-G, is also a potent opioid agonist and may accumulate in renal failure.

What to use morphine for
- Relief of severe pain.
- To facilitate mechanical ventilation.
- Acute left ventricular failure – by relieving anxiety and producing vasodilatation.

When not to use morphine
Airway obstruction
Pain caused by to biliary colic

How to use morphine
- IV bolus: 2.5 mg every 15 mins as necessary
- IV infusion rate: 1-5 mg/hr
  Dilute in 5% glucose or 0.9% saline
  Stop or reduce infusion each day and restart when first signs of discomfort appear. Failure to assess daily will result in overdosage and difficulty in weaning patient from ventilation.
- If the patient is conscious the best method is to give an infusion pump they can control (PCAS): 60 mg made up to 60 ml with 0.9% saline; IV bolus: 1 mg; lockout: 5-10 mins.

SYRINGE COMPATIBILITY
- Droperidol
- Metoclopramide

LINE COMPATIBILITY
- Atracurium
- Ondansetron
- Pancuronium
- Vecuronium

How not to use morphine
In combination with an opioid partial agonist e.g. buprenorphine (antagonises opioid effects).

Adverse effects

Respiratory depression and apnoea
Hypotension and tachycardia
Nausea and vomiting
Delayed gastric emptying
Reduced intestinal mobility
Biliary spasm
Constipation
Urinary retention
Histamine release
Tolerance
Pulmonary oedema

Cautions

Enhanced and prolonged effect when used in patients with renal failure, the elderly, and in patients with hypovolaemia and hypothermia.

Enhanced sedative and respiratory depression from interaction with:

• Benzodiazepines

• Antidepressants

• Antipsychotics

Head injury and neurosurgical patients (may exacerbate ↑ ICP as a result of ↑ $PaCO_2$)

Organ failure

CNS: Sedative effects increased
Respiratory: ↑ respiratory depression
Hepatic: Can precipitate coma
Renal: Increased cerebral sensitivity. M-6-G accumulates.

NALOXONE

This is a specific opioid antagonist. The elimination half-life is 60–90 mins, with a duration of action between 30-45 mins.

What to use naloxone for
- Reversal of opioid adverse effects – respiratory depression, sedation, pruritus and urinary retention.
- As a diagnostic test of opioid overdose in an unconscious patient.

When not to use naloxone
Patients physically dependent on opioids

How to use naloxone
- Reversal of opioid overdose: 200 µg IV bolus, repeat every 2-3 mins until desired response, up to a total of 2 mg.
- Reversal of spinal opioid induced pruritus: Dilute 200 µg in 10 ml WFI. Give 20 µg boluses every 5 mins until symptoms resolve.

Titrate dose carefully in postoperative patients to avoid sudden return of severe pain.

How not to use naloxone
Large doses given quickly

Adverse effects
Arrhythmias
Hypertension

Cautions
Withdrawal reactions in patients on long-term opioid for medical reasons or in addicts.
Postoperative patients – return of pain and severe haemodynamic disturbances (hypertension, VT/VF, pulmonary oedema).

Organ failure
Hepatic: Delayed elimination

PETHIDINE

Pethidine has one-tenth the analgesic potency of morphine. The duration of action is 2-4 hours. It has atropine-like actions and relaxes smooth muscles. The principle metabolite is norpethidine which can cause fits. In renal failure and after infusions this metabolite can accumulate and cause seizures.

What to use pethidine for

It may be indicated in controlling pain from pancreatitis, secondary to gallstones, and after a surgical procedure involving bowel anastomosis where it is claimed to cause less increase in the intraluminal pressures.

It produces less release of histamine than morphine, and may be preferable in asthmatics.

When not to use pethidine

Airway obstruction

How to use pethidine

IV bolus: 10 mg as necessary
PCAS: 600 mg in 60 ml 0.9% saline
            IV bolus: 10 mg, Lockout 5-10 mins

How not to use pethidine

In combination with an opioid partial agonist e.g. buprenorphine (antagonises opioid effects).

Adverse effects

Respiratory depression and apnoea
Hypotension and tachycardia
Nausea and vomiting
Delayed gastric emptying
Reduced intestinal mobility
Constipation
Urinary retention
Histamine release
Tolerance
Pulmonary oedema

Cautions

Enhanced sedative and respiratory depression from interaction with:

- Benzodiazepines.
- Antidepressants.
- Antipsychotics.

MAOI (hypertension, hyperpyrexia, convulsions and coma).
Head injury and neurosurgical patients (may exacerbate $\downarrow$ ICP as a result of $\uparrow PaCO_2$).

Organ failure

CNS: Sedative effects increased

Respiratory: $\uparrow$ respiratory depression

Hepatic: Enhanced and prolonged sedative effect.
Can precipitate coma.

Renal: Increased cerebral sensitivity.
Fits (norpethidine accumulates.)

ATRACURIUM

Atracurium is a non-depolarising neuromuscular blocker which is broken down by Hofmann degradation and ester hydrolysis. The ampoules have to be stored in the fridge to prevent spontaneous degradation. Atracurium has an elimination half-life of 20 mins. The principal metabolite is laudanosine which can cause convulsions in dogs. Even with long-term infusions, the concentration of laudanosine is well below the seizure threshold (17 µg/ml). It is the agent of choice in renal and hepatic failure.

What to use atracurium for
Muscle paralysis

When not to use atracurium
Airway obstruction
To facilitate tracheal intubation in patients at risk of regurgitation.

How to use atracurium
- IV bolus: 0.5 mg/kg, repeat with 0.15 mg/kg at 20-45 mins interval
- IV infusion: 0.2-0.4 mg/kg/hr

Monitor with peripheral nerve stimulator

LINE COMPATIBILITY
- Dopamine
- Fentanyl
- Midazolam
- Morphine

How not to use atracurium
As part of a rapid sequence induction
In the conscious patient
By persons not trained to intubate the trachea

Adverse effects
Bradycardia
Hypotension

Cautions
Asthmatics (histamine release)
Breathing circuit (disconnection)
Prolonged use (disuse muscle atrophy)

Organ failure
Hepatic: Increased concentration of laudanosine
Renal: Increased concentration of laudanosine

PANCURONIUM

A non–depolarising neuromuscular blocker with a long duration of action (1-2 hrs). It is largely excreted unchanged by the kidneys. It causes a 20% increase in HR and BP.

What to use pancuronium for
Patients where prolonged muscle relaxation is desirable e.g. intractable status asthmaticus.

Hypotensive patients, although the tachycardia induced may not be desirable if the HR is already high, e.g. hypovolaemia, septic shock.

When not to use pancuronium
Airway obstruction
To facilitate tracheal intubation in patients at risk of regurgitation
Renal and hepatic failure (prolonged paralysis)
Severe muscle atrophy
Tetanus (sympathomimetic effects)

How to use pancuronium
- Initial dose: 50-100 µg/kg IV
- Incremental doses: 20 µg/kg, every 1-2 hrs
Monitor with peripheral nerve stimulator

How not to use pancuronium
Do not mix with other drugs or dilute
As part of a rapid sequence induction
In the conscious patient
By persons not trained to intubate the trachea

Adverse effects
Tachycardia and hypertension

Cautions
Breathing circuit (disconnection)
Prolonged use (disuse muscle atrophy)

Organ failure
Hepatic: Prolonged paralysis
Renal: Prolonged paralysis

SUXAMETHONIUM

The only depolarising neuromuscular blocker available in the UK. It has a rapid onset of action (45-60 s) and a short duration of action (5 mins). Breakdown is dependent on plasma pseudocholinesterase. It is best to keep the ampoule in the fridge to prevent a gradual loss of activity caused by spontaneous hydrolysis.

What to use suxamethonium for

Agent of choice for:

- Rapid tracheal intubation as part of a rapid sequence induction.
- Procedures requiring short periods of muscle relaxation, e.g. electroconvulsive therapy.
- Management of severe post-extubation laryngospasm unresponsive to gentle positive pressure ventilation.

When not to use suxamethonium

History of malignant hyperpyrexia (potent trigger)

Hyperkalaemia (expect a further increase in K^+ level by 0.5-1.0 mmol/L)

Patients where an exaggerated increase in K^+ (>1.0 mmol/L) are expected:

- Severe burns.
- Extensive muscle damage.
- Disuse atrophy.
- Paraplegia and quadriplegia.
- Peripheral neuropathy e.g. Guillain-Barré.

How to use suxamethonium

- As a rapid sequence induction: 1-1.5 mg/kg IV bolus, after 3 mins preoxygenation with 100% O_2 and a sleep dose of induction agent (propofol 1.5-2.5 mg/kg or etomidate 2-3 mg/kg). Apply cricoid pressure until tracheal intubation confirmed. Intubation possible within 1 min. Effect normally lasting no more than 5 mins.
- Repeat dose of 0.25-0.5 mg/kg may be given. Atropine should be given at the same time to avoid bradycardia/asystole.

How not to use suxamethonium

In the conscious patient

By persons not trained to intubate the trachea

Adverse effects

Malignant hyperpyrexia

Hyperkalaemia

Transient increase in IOP and ICP

Muscle pain

Myotonia

Bradycardia, especially after repeated dose

Cautions

Digoxin (may cause arrhythmias)

Myasthenia gravis (resistant to usual dose)

Penetrating eye injury ($\uparrow$ IOP may cause loss of globe contents)

Prolonged block in:

- Patients taking aminoglycoside antibiotics, magnesium.

- Myathenic syndrome.

- Pseudocholinesterase deficiency (inherited or acquired).

Organ failure

Hepatic: Prolonged apnoea
(reduced synthesis of pseudocholinesterase)

VECURONIUM

A non-depolarising neuromuscular blocker with no cardiovascular effects. It is metabolised in the liver to inactive products and has a duration of action of 20-30 mins. Dose may have to be reduced in hepatic/renal failure.

What to use vecuronium for
Muscle paralysis

When not to use vecuronium
Airway obstruction
To facilitate tracheal intubation in patients at risk of regurgitation of stomach contents.

How to use vecuronium
Initial dose: 100 µg/kg IV
Incremental dose: 20-30 µg/kg according to response
Monitor with peripheral nerve stimulator

How not to use vecuronium
As part of a rapid sequence induction
In the conscious patient
By persons not trained to intubate the trachea

Cautions
Breathing circuit (disconnection)
Prolonged use (disuse muscle atrophy)

Organ failure
Hepatic: Prolonged duration of action
Renal: Prolonged duration of action

ANTICONVULSANTS

MANAGEMENT OF STATUS EPILEPTICUS

Status epilepticus is defined as continuous seizure activity lasting >30 mins. Many would have a previous history of fits. Other causes of status epilepticus are listed below.

CAUSES OF STATUS EPILEPTICUS

History of epilepsy
- Poor compliance with anticonvulsants
- Recent change in medication
- Drug interactions

No history of epilepsy
- Intracranial mass lesions
- Cerebral infarction
- Head injury or surgery
- Infection – meningitis, encephalitis
- Febrile convulsions in children
- Metabolic abnormalities – hypoglycaemia, hypocalcaemia, hyponatraemia, hypoxia
- Drug overdose
- Drug or alcohol withdrawal
- Use of antagonists in mixed drug overdoses

The aim of treatment is to stop the fitting and prevent further fits, but initial measures should be directed at supporting vital functions.

IV **diazepam** is the preferred first-line drug for stopping status epilepticus. However, it causes cardiorespiratory depression so it is not recommended in patients with acute neurological injury who are at risk of ↑ ICP. If IV access cannot be obtained diazepam may be given rectally. It takes up to 10 mins to work. The duration of action of diazepam in the brain is short (20–30 mins) because of rapid redistribution. This means that although a diazepam bolus is effective at stopping a fit, it will not prevent further fits.

Phenytoin should be started at the same time as giving diazepam to prevent further fits. Unlike diazepam it does not work immediately, taking 15-20 mins to reach peak concentration in the CSF. A loading dose should be given. Patients with known epilepsy may already be on phenytoin. Many of these patients will be having fits because of poor compliance. A lower loading dose should be given with the remainder given, if necessary, once the plasma phenytoin concentration is known.

If the patient has not responded to diazepam and phenytoin, **chlormethiazole** may be tried before proceeding to anaesthesia and ventilatory support. Chlormethiazole is particularly useful where fits are due to alcohol withdrawal.

Thiopentone is the favoured anaesthetic agent and many also use it at subanaesthetic doses. It has cerebroprotective action and potent anticonvulsant activity. The main disadvantages, however, are in its pharmacokinetics. Thiopentone has saturable kinetics, with a resultant long half-life at high concentrations. It has a tendency to accumulate, and it is not uncommon for a patient to remain comatose for days after stopping a relatively short thiopentone infusion. The favourable reports of subanaesthetic doses of thiopentone being used without ventilatory support should be interpreted cautiously and cannot be recommended.

TREATMENT OF STATUS EPILEPTICUS

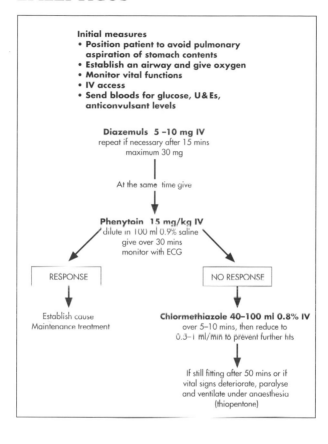

Initial measures
- **Position patient to avoid pulmonary aspiration of stomach contents**
- **Establish an airway and give oxygen**
- **Monitor vital functions**
- **IV access**
- **Send bloods for glucose, U & Es, anticonvulsant levels**

Diazemuls 5 –10 mg IV
repeat if necessary after 15 mins
maximum 30 mg

At the same time give

Phenytoin 15 mg/kg IV
dilute in 100 ml 0.9% saline
give over 30 mins
monitor with ECG

RESPONSE

Establish cause
Maintenance treatment

NO RESPONSE

Chlormethiazole 40–100 ml 0.8% IV
over 5–10 mins, then reduce to
0.3–1 ml/min to prevent further fits

If still fitting after 50 mins or if
vital signs deteriorate, paralyse
and ventilate under anaesthesia
(thiopentone)

CHLORMETHIAZOLE

The 0.8% solution for IV use contains only Na^+ 32 mmol/L and no other electrolytes. It has no analgesic effect, little cardiac and respiratory depression, and may be used in elderly patients.

What to use chlormethiazole for
Anticonvulsant

When not to use chlormethiazole
As it is only available in a dilute solution for IV use, it imposes a large waterload and should be avoided if there is fluid overload or cerebral/pulmonary oedema.

How to use chlormethiazole
IV infusion: 40-100 ml over 5-10 mins, then maintain at 0.5-1 ml/min according to response.

How not to use chlormethiazole
Rapid infusion (risk of apnoea and hypotension)
Prolonged use (risk of accumulation)
Abrupt withdrawal

Adverse effects
Increased nasopharyngeal and bronchial secretions
Thrombophlebitis
Tachycardia and transient decrease in BP

Cautions
Airway obstruction in deep sedation
Cardiac and respiratory disease – confusion may indicate hypoxia
Hepatic impairment – sedation can mask hepatic coma
Renal impairment

Organ failure
CNS: Risk of cerebral oedema
Cardiac: Risk of pulmonary oedema
Hepatic: Can precipitate coma
Renal: Increased cerebral sensitivity

DIAZEPAM

Available formulated in either propylene glycol or a lipid emulsion (diazemul) which causes minimal thrombophlebitis. Also available in a rectal solution (stesolid) which takes up to 10 mins to work.

What to use diazepam for
Ending of epileptic fit

When not to use diazepam
Airway obstruction

How to use diazepam
- IV: Diazemuls 5-10 mg over 2 mins, repeated if necessary after 15 mins, up to total 30 mg
- PR: Stesolid up to 20 mg

How not to use diazepam
IM injection - painful and unpredictable absorption

Adverse effects
Respiratory depression and apnoea
Drowsiness
Hypotension and bradycardia

Cautions
Airway obstruction with further neurological damage
Enhanced and prolonged sedative effect in the elderly
Additive effects with other CNS depressants

Organ failure
CNS: Enhanced and prolonged sedative effect
Respiratory: ↑ respiratory depression
Hepatic: Enhanced and prolonged sedative effect.
           Can precipitate coma.
Renal: Enhanced and prolonged sedative effect

MAGNESIUM SULPHATE

Magnesium sulphate has long been the mainstay of treatment for pre-eclampsia/eclampsia in America, but the practice in the UK until recently is to use more specific anti-convulsant and anti-hypertensive agents. A large international collaborative trial shows a lower risk of recurrent convulsions in eclamptic mothers given magnesium sulphate compared to those given diazepam or phenytoin.

Normal serum magnesium concentration: 0.7-1 mmol/L
Therapeutic range for pre-eclampsia/eclampsia: 2.0-3.5 mmol/L

What to use magnesium sulphate for
Preeclampsia
Anticonvulsant in eclampsia

When not to use magnesium sulphate
Hypocalcaemia (further $\downarrow Ca^{2+}$)
Heart block (risk of arrhythmias)

How to use magnesium sulphate
Magnesium sulphate solution for injection
1 g = 8 mEq = 4 mmol

Concentration %	g/ml	mEq/ml	mmol/ml
10	0.1	0.8	0.4
25	0.25	2	1
50	0.5	4	2

- Loading dose: 4 g (8 ml 50% solution) diluted in 250 ml 0.9% saline IV, over 10 mins.
- Maintenance: 1 g per hr IV, as necessary. Add 10 ml 50% magnesium sulphate to 40 ml 0.9% saline and infuse at 10 ml/hr.

Monitor: BP, respiratory rate
          ECG
          Tendon reflexes
          Renal function
          Serum magnesium level
Maintain urine output >30 ml/hr

How not to use magnesium sulphate
Rapid IV infusion can cause respiratory or cardiac arrest
IM injections (risk of abscess formation)

Adverse effects

Related to serum level:

4.0–6.5 mmol/L	Nausea and vomiting
	Somnolence
	Double vision
	Slurred speech
	Loss of patellar reflex
6.5–7.5 mmol/L	Muscle weakness and paralysis
	Respiratory arrest
	Bradycardia, arrhythmias and hypotension
>10 mmol/L	Cardiac arrest

Plasma concentrations >4.0 mmol/L cause toxicity which may be treated with calcium gluconate 1 g (10 ml 10%) IV.

Cautions

Oliguria and renal impairment (↑ risk of toxic levels)
Potentiates both depolarising and nondepolarising muscle relaxants
Newborn   monitor for hyperreflexia and respiratory depression

Organ failure

Renal: Reduce dose and slower infusion rate.
Closer monitoring for signs of toxicity.

PHENYTOIN

What to use phenytoin for
- Prevention and ending of grand mal and complex partial seizures
- Anticonvulsant prophylaxis after neurosurgical operations.
- Antiarrhythmic – particularly for arrhythmias associated with digoxin toxicity.

When not to use phenytoin
Do not use IV phenytoin in sinoatrial block, or second- and third-degree AV block

How to use phenytoin
- Status epilepticus: 15 mg/kg in 100 ml 0.9% saline IV, over 30 mins, followed by 100 mg every 6-8 hrly.
- Anticonvulsant prophylaxis: 200-600 mg/day orally/IV.
- Antiarrhythmic: 100 mg in 50 ml 0.9% saline IV every 15 mins until arrhythmia stops. Maximum 15 mg/kg/day.

Monitor: ECG and BP
          Serum phenytoin level (p 9)

How not to use phenytoin
Rapid IV (severe hypotension or CNS depression)
Do not dissolve in solutions containing glucose (precipitation)
Do not give into an artery (gangrene)

Adverse effects
Nystagmus, ataxia and slurred speech
Drowsiness and confusion
Hypotension (rapid IV)
Rashes
Aplastic anaemia
Agranulocytosis
Megaloblastic anaemia
Thrombocytopenia

Cautions
Severe liver disease (reduce dose)
Metabolism subject to other enzyme inducers and inhibitors (p 7)
Additive CNS depression with other CNS depressants

Organ failure
CNS: Enhanced sedation
Hepatic: Increased serum concentration

THIOPENTONE

The most widely used IV anaesthetic agent. It is an anaesthetically active barbiturate which also has cerebroprotective and anticonvulsant activitivies. Awakening from a bolus dose is rapid due to redistribution, but hepatic metabolism is slow and sedative effects may persist for 24 hrs. Repeated doses or infusion have a cumulative effect. Available in 500 mg ampoules or 2.5 g vial which is dissolved in 20 ml or 100 ml WFI respectively to make a 2.5% solution.

What to use thiopentone for
Induction of anaesthesia
Status epilepticus

When not to use thiopentone
Airway obstruction
Previous hypersensitivity
Status asthmaticus
Porphyria

How to use thiopentone
IV bolus: 2.5–4 mg/kg. After injecting a test dose of 2 ml, if no pain, give the rest over 20–30 s until loss of eyelash reflex. Give further 50–100 mg if necessary.

Reduce dose and inject more slowly in the elderly, patients with severe hepatic and renal impairment, and in hypovolaemic and shocked patients.

In obese patients, dosage should be based on lean body mass

How not to use thiopentone
Intra-arterial injection (pain and ischaemic damage)
Do not inject solution > 2.5% (thrombophlebitis)

Adverse effects
Hypersensitivity reactions (1:14 000 – 1:35 000)
Coughing, laryngospasm
Bronchospasm (histamine release)
Respiratory depression and apnoea
Hypotension, myocardial depression
Tachycardia, arrhythmias
Tissue necrosis from extravasation

Cautions
Hypovolaemia
Septic shock
Elderly (reduce dose)

Organ failure
CNS: Sedative effects increased
Cardiac: Exaggerated hypotension and ↓ cardiac output
Respiratory: ↑ respiratory depression
Hepatic: Enhanced and prolonged sedative effect.
              Can precipitate coma.
Renal: Increased cerebral sensitivity

CARDIOVASCULAR DRUGS

ANTI-ARRHYTHMIC DRUGS

The traditional Vaughan Williams' classification (based on electro-physiological action) does not include anti-arrhythmic drugs such as digoxin and atropine. A more clinically useful classification categorises drugs according to the cardiac tissues which each affects, and may be of use when a choice is to be made to treat an arrhythmia arising from that part of the heart.

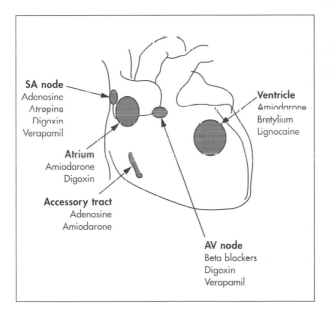

SA node
Adenosine
Atropine
Digoxin
Verapamil

Ventricle
Amiodarone
Bretylium
Lignocaine

Atrium
Amiodarone
Digoxin

Accessory tract
Adenosine
Amiodarone

AV node
Beta blockers
Digoxin
Verapamil

ADENOSINE

This endogenous nucleoside is safe and effective in ending over 90% of paroxysmal SVTs. After an IV bolus effects are immediate (10-30 s), dose related, and transient (half life <10 s; entirely eliminated from plasma in <1 min, being degraded by vascular endothelium and erythrocytes). Its elimination is not affected by renal/hepatic disease. Adenosine works faster and is superior to verapamil. It may be used in cardiac failure, in hypotension, and with beta-blockers, in all of which verapamil is contraindicated.

What to use adenosine for

It has both therapeutic and diagnostic uses.

- Alternative to DC cardioversion in terminating paroxysmal SVT, including those associated with WPW syndrome.
- Determining the origin of broad complex tachycardia; SVT responds, VT does not (predictive accuracy 92%; partly because VT may occasionally respond). Though adenosine does no harm in VT, verapamil may produce hypotension or cardiac arrest.

What not to use adenosine for

Atrial flutter or AF
Second or third degree heart block (unless pacemaker fitted)
Sick sinus syndrome (unless pacemaker fitted)

How to use adenosine

3 mg over 1-2 s into a large vein, followed by rapid flushing with 0.9% saline.
If no effect after 1-2 mins give 6 mg. Repeat if needed at 12 mg.

Need continuous ECG monitoring
More effective given via a central vein or into right atrium

How not to use adenosine

Without continuous ECG monitor

Adverse effects

Flushing (18%), dyspnoea (12%), and chest discomfort are the commonest side effects but are well tolerated and invariably last <1 min.

Cautions

Atrial fibrillation or flutter with accessory pathway ($\uparrow$ conduction down anomalous pathway may develop)

Early relapse of paroxysmal SVT is more common than with verapamil but usually responds to further dose.

Asthmatic   –   may cause bronchospasm

                –   if taking theophylline preparation, may need higher doses (antagonised by methylxanthines)

Dipyridamole potentiates adenosine's effect – reduce dose (start with 0.5 mg)

AMIODARONE

Amiodarone has a broad spectrum of activity on the heart. In addition to having anti-arrhythmic activity, it also has anti-anginal effects. This may result from its alpha- and beta-adrenoceptor blocking properties as well as from its calcium channel blocking effect in the coronary vessels. It causes minimal myocardial depression. It is therefore often a first-line drug in critical care situations. It has an extremely long half-life (15-105 days). Unlike oral amiodarone, IV administration usually acts relatively rapidly (20-30 mins).

What to use amiodarone for

Good results with both ventricular and supraventricular arrhythmias, including those associated with Wolff-Parkinson-White syndrome.

When not to use amiodarone

Iodine sensitivity (amiodarone contains iodine)
Sinus bradycardia (risk of asystole)
Heart block (unless pacemaker fitted)

How to use amiodarone

Loading: 300 mg in 250 ml 5% dextrose IV over 20-120 mins, followed by a dose of 900 mg in 500 ml 5% dextrose over 24 hrs.
Maintenance: 600 mg IV/PO daily for 7 days, then 200 mg IV/PO daily.

Administer IV via central line

Continuous cardiac monitoring

How not to use amiodarone

Incompatible with 0.9% saline
Do not use peripheral vein (thrombophlebitis)

Adverse effects

Short term
- Skin reactions common.
- Vasodilation and hypotension or bradycardia after rapid infusion.
- Corneal microdeposits (reversible on stopping).
- Nightmares

Long term
- Pulmonary fibrosis, alveolitis and pneumonitis (reversible on stopping).
- Liver dysfunction (asymptomatic ↑ in LFTs common).

- Hypo- or hyperthyroidism (check TFTs before starting drug).
- Peripheral neuropathy, myopathy and cerebellar dysfunction (reversible on stopping).

Cautions

Increased risk of bradycardia, AV block and myocardial depression with beta-blockers and calcium-channel antagonists.

Potentiates the effect of digoxin, theophylline and warfarin - reduce dose.

Organ failure

Respiratory: Bronchospasm and apnoea
Hepatic: Worsens
Renal: Accumulation of iodine may ↑ risk of thyroid dysfunction

ATROPINE

The influence of atropine is most noticeable in healthy young adults in whom vagal tone is considerable. In infancy and old age, even large doses may fail to accelerate the heart.

What to use atropine for
Asystole (p 15)
Sinus bradycardia – will increase BP as a result
Reversal of muscarinic effects of anticholinesterases (neostigmine)
Organophosphate poisoning

When not to use atropine
Complete heart block
Tachycardia

How to use atropine
- Bradycardia: 0.3-1 mg IV bolus, up to 3 mg (total vagolytic dose), may be diluted with WFI
- Asystole: 3 mg IV bolus, once only (see algorithm p 15)
- Reversal of muscarinic effects of anticholinesterase: 1.2 mg for every 2.5 mg neostigmine
- Organophosphate poisoning: 1-2 mg initially, then further 1-2 mg every 30 mins as required

How not to use atropine
Slow IV injection of doses < 0.3 mg (bradycardia caused by medullary vagal stimulation)

Adverse effects
Drowsiness, confusion
Dry mouth
Blurred vision
Urinary retention
Tachycardia
Pyrexia (suppression of sweating)
Atrial arrhythmias and atrioventricular dissociation (without significant cardiovascular symptoms)

Dose >5 mg results in restlessness and excitation, hallucinations, delirium and coma.

Cautions

Elderly (↑ CNS side-effects)

Child with pyrexia (further ↑ temperature)

Acute myocardial ischaemia or MI (tachycardia may cause worsening)

Prostatic hypertrophy – urinary retention (unless patient catheterised)

Paradoxically, bradycardia may occur at low doses (< 0.3 mg)

Acute-angle glaucoma (further ↑ IOP)

Pregnancy (fetal tachycardia)

DIGOXIN

A cardiac glycoside with both anti-arrhythmic and inotropic properties. It is principally excreted unchanged by the kidney and will therefore accumulate in renal impairment.

What to use digoxin for

Supraventricular tachycardias, especially for controlling ventricular response in AF and atrial flutter.
Heart failure may also be improved, even in patients in sinus rhythm.

When not to use digoxin

Intermittent complete heart block
Second degree AV block
Wolff-Parkinson-White syndrome
Hypertrophic obstructive cardiomyopathy
Constrictive pericarditis

How to use digoxin

- IV loading dose: 0.5–1 mg in 50 ml 5% dextrose or 0.9% saline, over 2 hrs
- Maintenance dose: 62.5–500 µg daily (renal function is the most important determinant of maintenance dosage)

Monitor: ECG
Serum digoxin level (p 9)

How not to use digoxin

IM injections

Adverse effects

Anorexia, nausea, vomiting
Diarrhoea, abdominal pain
Visual disturbances, headache
Fatigue, drowsiness, confusion, delirium, hallucinations
Arrhythmias – all forms
Heart block

Cautions

Absorption from oral administration reduced by sucralfate and ion-exchange resins, cholestyramine and colestipol.

Hypokalaemia and hypomagnesaemia increases the sensitivity to digoxin, and the following drugs may predispose to toxicity:

- Amphotericin
- β_2 sympathomimetics
- Corticosteroids
- Loop diuretics
- Thiazides

Hypercalcaemia is inhibitory to the positive inotropic action of digoxin and potentiates the toxic effects.

Plasma concentration of digoxin increased by:

- Amiodarone
- Diltiazem
- Nicardipine
- Propafenone
- Quinidine
- Verapamil

Digoxin toxicity (DC shock may cause fatal ventricular arrhythmia) – stop digoxin at least 24 hrs prior to cardioversion.

Beta-blockers and verapamil increase AV block and bradycardia.

Suxamethonium predisposes to arrhythmias.

Organ failure

Renal: Toxicity – reduce dose

ISOPRENALINE

Isoprenaline is a β_1 and β_2 adrenoceptor agonist causing: ↑ HR, ↑ automaticity, ↑ contractility, ↓ diastolic BP, ↑ systolic BP, ↑ myocardial oxygen demand and bronchodilation. It has a half–life of <5 mins.

What to use isoprenaline for
Complete heart block, whilst getting temporary pacing established

What not to use isoprenaline for
Tachyarrhythmias
Heart block caused by digoxin

How to use isoprenaline
IV infusion: up to 20 µg/min
4 mg made up to 50 ml 5% dextrose (80 µg/ml)

Dose (µg/min)	Infusion rate (ml/hr)
1	0.75
2	1.5
4	3
10	7.5
20	15

How not to use isoprenaline
Do not use 0.9% saline as a diluent

Adverse effects
Tachycardia
Arrhythmias
Angina
Hypotension

Cautions
Risk of arrythmias with concurrent use of other sympathomimetics and volatile anaesthetics.

LIGNOCAINE

This anti-arrhythmic agent suppresses automaticity of conduction and spontaneous depolarisation of the ventricles during diastole. Clearance is related to both hepatic blood flow and function; it will be prolonged in liver disease, cardiac failure and in the elderly. The effects after the first bolus dose last approximately 20 mins. An IV infusion is needed to maintain the anti-arrhythmic effect.

What to use lignocaine for
Prevention of ventricular ectopic beats, VT and VF after MI

What not to use lignocaine for
It is no longer the first-line drug in pulseless VT or VF during a cardiac arrest
Hypersensitivity to amide-type local anaesthetics (rare)
Heart block (risk of asystole)

How to use lignocaine
- Loading dose: 1.5 mg/kg IV over 2 mins, repeat after 5 mins to a total dose of 3 mg/kg if necessary. Reduce dose in the elderly.
- Maintenance dose: 4 mg/min for 1st hr
  2 mg/min for 2nd hr
  1 mg/min thereafter

Reduce infusion rates in patients with hepatic impairment, cardiac failure and in the elderly.

Undiluted 40 ml 2 % solution (800 mg)
  4 mg/min = 12 ml/hr
  2 mg/min = 6 ml/hr
  1 mg/min = 3 ml/hr

Monitor: ECG
  BP

How not to use lignocaine
Rapid IV bolus (should not be given at a rate >50 mg/min)

Adverse effects
Paraesthesia, muscle twitching, tinnitus
Anxiety, drowsiness, confusion, convulsions
Hypotension, bradycardia, asystole

Cautions

Elderly (reduced volume of distribution, reduce dose by 50%)
Hepatic impairment
Cardiac failure
Other class 1 anti-arrhythmics e.g. phenytoin, may increase risk of toxicity

Organ failure

Cardiac: Reduce dose
Hepatic: Reduce dose

MAGNESIUM SULPHATE

Like potassium, magnesium is one of the major cations of the body responsible for neurotransmission and neuromuscular excitability. Regulation of magnesium balance is mainly by the kidneys. Hypomagnesaemia should be suspected in association with other fluid and electrolyte disturbances when the patient develops unexpected neurological features or cardiac arrhythmias.
Normal range: 0.7-1 mmol/L

What to use magnesium sulphate for
Hypomagnesaemia associated with cardiac arrhythmias

When not to use magnesium sulphate
Hypocalcaemia (further $\downarrow$ Ca^{2+})
Heart block (risk of arrhythmias)

How to use magnesium sulphate
Magnesium sulphate solution for injection
1 g = 8 mEq = 4 mmol

Concentration %	g/ml	mEq/ml	mmol/ml
10	0.1	0.8	0.4
25	0.25	2	1
50	0.5	4	2

IV infusion: 20 mmol diluted in 100 ml 5% dextrose, given over 1 hr
Do not give at a rate >30 mmol/hr
Repeat until plasma level is normal
Concentrations <20% are suitable for peripheral IV administration
Monitor: BP, respiratory rate
          ECG
          Tendon reflexes
          Renal function
          Serum magnesium level
Maintain urine output >30 ml/hr

How not to use magnesium sulphate
Rapid IV infusion (respiratory or cardiac arrest)
IM injections (risk of abscess formation)

CARDIOVASCULAR DRUGS
MAGNESIUM SULPHATE

Adverse effects

Related to serum level:

4.0–6.5 mmol/L	Nausea and vomiting
	Somnolence
	Double vision
	Slurred speech
	Loss of patellar reflex
6.5–7.5 mmol/L	Muscle weakness and paralysis
	Respiratory arrest
	Bradycardia, arrhythmias and hypotension
>10 mmol/L	Cardiac arrest

Cautions

Oliguria and renal impairment ($\uparrow$ risk of toxic levels)

Organ failure

Renal: Reduce dose and slower infusion rate. Closer monitoring for signs of toxicity.

VERAPAMIL

A calcium channel blocker which prolongs the refractory period of the AV node.

What to use verapamil for
SVT
AF
Atrial flutter

What not to use verapamil for
Sinus bradycardia
Heart block
Congestive cardiac failure
VT/VF – may produce severe hypotension or cardiac arrest
Wolff–Parkinson–White syndrome

How to use verapamil
- IV bolus: 5–10 mg over 2 mins, may repeat with 10 mg in 30 mins
- IV infusion: 0.3 mg/kg/hr
  Decrease dose in: liver disease, elderly

Monitor: ECG
        BP

How not to use verapamil
In combination with beta-blockers (bradycardia, heart failure, asystole)

Adverse effects
Bradycardia
Hypotension
Heart block
Asystole

Cautions
Sick sinus syndrome
Hypertrophic obstructive cardiomyopathy
Severe hypotension may occur with fentanyl
Increased risk of toxicity from theophylline and digoxin

Organ failure
Hepatic: Reduce dose

INOTROPES AND VASOPRESSORS

Which inotrope to choose?

Inotropes should be used only after the intravascular volume has been restored to an adequate level. If intravascular volume has been restored (PCWP 10-15 mmHg) but perfusion is still inadequate, the selection should be based on the ability of the drug to correct or augment the haemodynamic deficit. If the problem is felt to be inadequate cardiac output, the drug chosen should have prominent activity at beta-1 receptors and little alpha activity which would increase afterload and further reduce stroke volume. If the perfusion deficit is caused by a marked reduction in SVR, then a drug with alpha activity should be used.

The haemodynamic picture is often more complex that those presented above. Other special considerations such as oliguria, underlying ischaemic heart disease, or arrhythmias may exist and affect the choice of drug.

Adrenaline is useful when there is severe reductions in cardiac output in whom the arrhythmogenecity and marked increase in HR and myocardial oxygen consumption that occur with this drug are not limiting factors. It is the drug of choice in anaphylactic shock, due to its activity at β_1 and β_2 receptors and its stabilising effect on mast cells.

Dopamine is also useful in hypoperfusion caused by a reduced cardiac output. It causes less of an increase in myocardial oxygen consumption than adrenaline. A further advantage is its ability to increase mesenteric and renal blood flow plus urine output at low doses. Dopamine tends to cause more tachycardia than dobutamine and unlike dobutamine usually increases rather than decreases pulmonary artery pressure and PCWP. At high doses it can increase SVR, but may be less reliable than noradrenaline. If dopamine fails to restore BP at 20 µg/kg/min, noradrenaline should be used.

Noradrenaline is used to restore BP in cases of reduced SVR. It can be used to good effect in septic shock when combined with dobutamine to optimise oxygen delivery and consumption.

Dobutamine is used when the reduced cardiac output is considered the cause of the perfusion deficit, and should not be used as the sole agent if the decrease in output is accompanied by a significant decrease in BP. This is because dobutamine causes reductions in preload and afterload which further reduce the BP.

The current interest in **dopexamine** is centred on its dopaminergic and anti-inflammatory activity. In critically ill patients it improves splanchnic blood flow.

The phosphodiesterase III inhibitors, **enoximone** and **milrinone** are both potent inodilators, and because they do not act via adrenergic receptors, they may be effective when catecholamines have failed. They may also show synergy with catecholamines and have the added advantage of causing less ↑ myocardial oxygen consumption. In septic shock there is a significant risk of hypotension and they should not be used. Nevertheless it is possible to ↑ both CO and MAP in patients with septic shock when used alone or in combination with adrenaline. Their major indication is in the short-term treatment of severe congestive heart failure unresponsive to conventional therapy.

INOTROPES: RECEPTORS STIMULATED

Drug	Dose: µg/kg/min	alpha 1	beta 1	beta 2	DA1
Dopamine	1-5				++
	5-10		+	+	++
	> 10	+	+	+	++
Dobutamine	1-25	0/+	+	+	
Dopexamine	0.5-6		0/+	++++	+
Adrenaline	0.01-0.2	+/++	+	+	
Noradrenaline	0.01-0.2	+++	+		

EFFECTS OF INOTROPES

Drug	Cardiac contractility	Heart rate	SVR	Blood pressure	Renal and mesenteric blood flow
Dopamine:					
DA 1	0	0	0	0	+
beta	++	+	0/+	+	0
alpha	0	0	++	++	−
Dobutamine	++	0	−	+	0
Dopexamine	0/+	+	−	0	0
Adrenaline	++	+	+/−	+	0/−
Noradrenaline	+	−	++	++	−

+ increase
0 no change
− decrease

ADRENALINE

Both α- and β- adrenergic receptors are stimulated. Low doses tend to produce predominantly α-effects whilst higher doses tend to produce predominantly β-effects. Stimulation of β_1-receptors in the heart increases the rate and force of contraction, resulting in an increase in cardiac output. Stimulation of α_1-receptor causes peripheral vasoconstriction, which increases the systolic BP. Stimulation of α_2-receptors causes bronchodilation and vasodilation in certain vascular beds. Consequently, total systemic resistance may actually decrease, explaining the decrease in diastolic pressure that is sometimes seen.

What to use adrenaline for
Low cardiac output states
Cardiac arrest (p 13)
Anaphylaxis (p 18)

When not to use adrenaline
Before adequate intravascular volume replacement

How to use adrenaline
• Low cardiac output states
Dose: 0.01-0.2 μg/kg/min IV infusion via a central vein
Titrate dose according to HR, BP, CVP, PCWP, cardiac output, presence of ectopic beats and urine output

4 mg made up to 50 ml 5% dextrose (80 μg/ml)

Dosage chart: ml/hr

Weight: kg	Dose: μg/kg/min				
	0.02	0.05	0.1	0.15	0.2
50	0.8	1.9	3.8	5.6	7.5
60	0.9	2.3	4.5	6.8	9
70	1.1	2.6	5.3	7.9	10.5
80	1.2	3	6	9	12
90	1.4	3.4	6.8	10.1	13.5
100	1.5	3.8	7.5	11.3	15
110	1.7	4.1	8.3	12.4	16.5
120	1.8	4.5	9	13.5	18

How not to use adrenaline

In the absence of haemodynamic monitoring

Do not connect to CVP lumen used for monitoring pressure (surge of drug during flushing of line).

Adverse effects

Arrhythmia

Tachycardia

Hypertension

Myocardial ischaemia

Cautions

Acute myocardial ischaemia or MI

DOBUTAMINE

A β_1 agonist that increases heart rate and force of contraction. It also has mild β_2- and α_1-effects and decreases peripheral and pulmonary vascular resistance. Systolic BP may be increased because of the augmented cardiac output.

What to use dobutamine for
Short-term management of heart failure
Septic shock

When not to use dobutamine for
Before adequate intravascular volume replacement
Idiopathic hypertrophic subaortic stenosis

How to use dobutamine
1-25 µg/kg/min IV infusion via a central vein
Titrate dose according to HR, BP, CVP, PCWP, cardiac output, presence of ectopic beats and urine output

250 mg made up to 50 ml 5% dextrose or 0.9% saline (5000 µg/ml)

Dosage chart: ml/hr

Weight: kg	Dose. µg/kg/min					
	2.5	5.0	7.5	10	15	20
50	1.5	3	4.5	6	9	12
60	1.8	3.6	5.4	7.2	10.8	14.5
70	2.1	4.2	6.3	8.4	12.75	16.8
80	2.4	4.8	7.2	9.6	14.4	19.2
90	2.7	5.4	8.1	10.8	16.2	21.6
100	3	6	9	12	18	24
110	3.3	6.6	9.9	13.2	19.85	26.4
120	3.6	7.2	10.8	14.4	21.6	28.8

LINE COMPATIBILITY
Atracurium
Calcium chloride/gluconate
Dopamine
Magnesium sulphate
Pancuronium
Potassium chloride
Vecuronium

How not use dobutamine
No invasive cardiac monitoring
Inadequate correction of hypovolaemia before starting dobutamine
Do not mix with sodium bicarbonate, frusemide or other alkaline solutions

Adverse effects
Tachycardia
Ectopic beats

Cautions
Acute myocardial ischaemia or MI
Beta-blockers (may cause dobutamine to be less effective)

DOPAMINE

A naturally occurring catecholamine that acts directly on α, β_1 and dopaminergic receptors and indirectly by releasing noradrenaline.

- At low doses (0.5-2.5 µg/kg/min) it increases renal and mesenteric blood flow by stimulating dopamine receptors. The ↑ renal blood flow results in ↑ GFR and ↑ renal sodium excretion.
- Doses of 2.5-10 µg/kg/min stimulate β_1-receptors causing ↑ myocardial contractility, stroke volume and cardiac output.
- Doses >10 µg/kg/min stimulate α-receptors causing ↑ SVR, ↓ renal blood flow and ↑ potential for arrhythmias.

What to use dopamine for
- Low dose to maintain urine output
- Septic shock
- Low cardiac output

What not to use dopamine for
- Attempt to increase urine output in patients inadequately resuscitated
- Phaeochromocytoma
- Tachyarrhythmias or VF

How to use dopamine
- Low dose: 0.5-2.5 µg/kg/min to produce a diuresis.
- Larger doses: 2.5-10 µg/kg/min to increase cardiac contractility
- Doses >10 µg/kg/min stimulates α-receptors and may cause renal vasoconstriction

200 mg made up to 50 ml 5% dextrose or 0.9% saline (4000 µg/ml)

Dosage chart: ml/hr

Weight: kg	Dose: µg/kg/min				
	2.5	5.0	7.5	10	15
50	1.9	3.8	5.6	7.5	11.3
60	2.3	4.5	6.8	9	13.5
70	2.6	5.3	7.9	10.5	15.8
80	3	6	9	12	18
90	3.4	6.8	10.1	13.5	20.3
100	3.8	7.5	11.3	15	22
110	4.1	8.3	12.4	16.5	24.8
120	4.5	9	13.5	18	27

Give via a central vein using an accurate infusion pump.
Reduce dosage if urine output decreases or there is increasing tachycardia or development of new arrhythmias.

LINE COMPATIBILITY
- Atracurium
- Dobutamine
- Morphine
- Potassium chloride
- Pancuronium
- Vecuronium

How not to use dopamine

Do not use a peripheral vein (risk of extravasation).
Do not connect to CVP lumen used for monitoring pressure (surge of drug during flushing of line).
Do not mix with sodium bicarbonate, frusemide or other alkaline solutions (dopamine inactivated).
Discard solution if cloudy, discoloured, or >24 hr old.

Adverse effects

Ectopic beats
Tachycardia
Angina
Gut ischaemia
Vasoconstriction

Cautions

MAOI (reduce dose by one–tenth of usual dose).
Peripheral vascular disease (monitor any changes in colour or temperature of the skin of the extremities).
If extravasation of dopamine occurs – Phentolamine 10 mg in 15 ml 0.9% saline should be infiltrated into the ischaemic area with a 23 G needle.

Organ failure

May accumulate in septic shock because of ↓ hepatic function

DOPEXAMINE

What to use dopexamine for
To improve renal, mesenteric, splanchnic and hepatic blood flow
Short-term treatment of acute heart failure

When not to use dopexamine
Concurrent MAOI administration
Left ventricular outlet obstruction (HOCM, aortic stenosis)
Phaeochromocytoma

How to use dopexamine
Correction of hypovolaemia before starting dopexamine
Dose: Start at 0.5 µg/kg/min, increasing up to 6 µg/kg/min
Titrate according to patient's response: HR, rhythm, BP, urine output and, whenever possible, cardiac output.

200 mg made up to 50 ml 5% dextrose or 0.9% saline (4000 µg/ml)

Dosage chart: ml/hr

Weight: kg	Dose: µg/kg/min						
	0.5	1	2	3	4	5	6
50	0.4	0.8	1.5	2.3	3	3.8	4.5
60	0.5	0.9	1.8	2.7	3.6	4.5	5.4
70	0.5	1.1	2.1	3.2	4.2	5.3	6.3
80	0.6	1.2	2.4	3.6	4.8	6	7.2
90	0.7	1.4	2.7	4.1	5.4	6.8	8.1
100	0.8	1.5	3	4.5	6	7.5	9
110	0.8	1.7	3.3	5	6.6	8.3	9.9
120	0.9	1.8	3.6	5.4	7.2	9	10.8

How not to use dopexamine
In patients with markedly reduced SVR (further reduction)
Do not add to sodium bicarbonate

Adverse effects
Dose-related increases in HR
Hypotension
Angina
Hypokalaemia
Hyperglycaemia

Cautions
Thrombocytopenia (a further decrease may occur)
IHD (especially following acute MI)

ENOXIMONE

Enoximone is a selective phosphodiesterase III inhibitor resulting in ↑ CO, and ↓ PCWP and SVR, without a significant ↑ in HR and myocardial oxygen consumption. It has a long half-life and haemodynamic effects can persist for 8-10 hrs after the drug is stopped.

What to use enoximone for
Severe congestive cardiac failure
Low cardiac output states (+/− dobutamine)

What not to use enoximone for
Severe aortic or pulmonary stenosis (exaggerated hypotension)
Hypertrophic obstructive cardiomyopathy (exaggerated hypotension)

How to use enoximone
- IV infusion: 0.5-1 mg/kg , then 5-20 µg/kg/min maintenance
  Available in 20 ml ampoules containing 100 mg enoximone
  (5 mg/ml)

  Dilute this 20 ml solution with 20 ml 0.9% saline giving a solution containing enoximone 2.5 mg/ml.

Total dose in 24 hrs should not >24 mg/kg

How not to use enoximone
Very alkaline solution (incompatible with all catecholamines in solution)
5% dextrose or contact with glass may result in crystal formation

Adverse effects
Hypotension
Arrhythmias

Cautions
In septic shock enoximone can cause prolonged hypotension

MILRINONE

Milrinone is a selective phosphodiesterase III inhibitor resulting in ↑ CO, and ↓ PCWP and SVR, without a significant ↑ in HR and myocardial oxygen consumption. It produces slight enhancement in AV node conduction and may ↑ ventricular rate in uncontrolled AF/atrial flutter.

What to use milrinone for
Severe congestive cardiac failure

What not to use milrinone for
Severe aortic or pulmonary stenosis (exaggerated hypotension)
Hypertrophic obstructive cardiomyopathy (exaggerated hypotension)

How to use milrinone
IV infusion: 50 µg/kg loading dose over 10 mins, then maintain on 0.375-0.75 µg/kg/min to a maximum haemodynamic effect.
Available in 10 ml ampoules containing 10 mg milrinone (1 mg/ml)
Dilute this 10 ml solution with 40 ml 0.9% saline or 5% dextrose giving a solution containing milrinone 200 µg/ml

Dose (µg/kg/min)	Infusion rate (ml/kg/hr)
0.375	0.11
0.4	0.12
0.5	0.15
0.6	0.18
0.7	0.21
0.75	0.22

Maximum daily dose: 1.13 mg/kg

In renal impairment:

CC (ml/min)	Dose (µg/kg/min)
20 - 50	0.28 0.43
10 - 20	0.23 - 0.28
<10	0.2 - 0.23

Adjustment of the infusion rate should be made according to haemodynamic response.

How not to use milrinone

Frusemide and bumetanide should not be given in the same line as milrinone (precipitation)

Adverse effects

Hypotension
Arrhythmias

Cautions

Uncontrolled AF/atrial flutter

Organ failure

Renal: Reduce dose

NORADRENALINE

Alpha-1 effect predominates over its beta-1 effect, increasing the BP by increasing the SVR. It increases the myocardial oxygen requirement without increasing coronary blood flow. Noradrenaline reduces renal, hepatic, and muscle blood flow.

What to use noradrenaline for
Septic shock, with low SVR

When not to use noradrenaline
Hypovolaemic shock
Acute myocardial ischaemia or MI

How to use noradrenaline
• IV infusion: 0.01–0.2 µg/kg/min via a central vein.
Start at a high rate than intended to increase the BP rapidly and then reduce rate

4 mg made up to 50 ml 5% dextrose (80 µg/ml)

Dosage chart: ml/hr

Weight: kg	Dose: µg/kg/min				
	0.02	0.05	0.1	0.15	0.2
50	0.8	1.9	3.8	5.6	7.5
60	0.9	2.3	4.5	6.8	9
70	1.1	2.6	5.3	7.9	10.5
80	1.2	3	6	9	12
90	1.4	3.4	6.8	10.1	13.5
100	1.5	3.8	7.5	11.3	15
110	1.7	4.1	8.3	12.4	16.5
120	1.8	4.5	9	13.5	18

How not to use noradrenaline
In the absence of haemodynamic monitoring
Do not use a peripheral vein (risk of extravasation)
Do not connect to CVP lumen used for monitoring pressure (surge of drug during flushing of line)

Adverse effects

Bradycardia

Hypertension

Arrhythmias

Myocardial ischaemia

Cautions

Hypertension

Heart disease

If extravasation of noradrenaline occurs – Phentolamine 10 mg in 15 ml 0.9% saline should be infiltrated into the ischaemic area with a 23 G needle.

HYPOTENSIVE DRUGS

HYDRALAZINE

Hydralazine lowers the BP by reducing arterial resistance through a direct relaxation of arteriolar smooth muscle. This effect is limited by reflex tachycardia and is best combined with a beta–blocker. Metabolism occurs by hepatic acetylation, the rate of which is genetically determined. Fast acetylators show a reduced therapeutic effect until the enzyme system is saturated.

What to use hydralazine for
All grades of hypertension
Pre-eclampsia

What not to use hydralazine for
Systemic lupus erythematosus
Dissecting aortic aneurysm
Right ventricular failure due to pulmonary hypertension (corpulmonale)
Severe tachycardia and heart failure with a high cardiac output state e.g. thyrotoxicosis
Severe aortic outflow obstruction (aortic stenosis, mitral stenosis, constrictive pericarditis)

How to use hydralazine
- IV bolus: 10-20 mg over 3-5 mins
  Reconstitute the ampoule containing 20 mg powder with 1 ml WFI, further dilute with 10 ml 0.9% saline, give over 3-5 mins.
  Expect to see response after 20 mins
  Repeat after 20-30 mins as necessary
- IV infusion: 2-15 mg/hr
  Reconstitute 3 ampoules (60 mg) of hydralazine with 1 ml WFI each. Make up to 60 mls with 0.9% saline (1mg/ml)
  Give at a rate between 2-15 mg/hr depending on the BP and pulse

Rapid acetylators may require higher doses

How not to use hydralazine
Do not dilute in fluids containing dextrose (glucose causes breakdown of hydralazine)

Adverse effects

Headache

Tachycardia

Hypotension

Myocardial ischaemia

Sodium and fluid retention, producing oedema and reduced urinary volume (prevented by concomitant use of a diuretic).

Lupus erythematosus (commoner slow acetylator status, women, and if treatment >6 months at doses >100 mg daily).

Cautions

Cerebrovascular disease

Cardiac disease (angina, immediately post MI)

Use with other antihypertensives and nitrate drugs may produce additive hypotensive effects.

Organ failure

Hepatic: Prolonged effect

Renal: Increased hypotensive effect (start with small dose)

LABETALOL

Labetalol is a combined α- and β-adrenoceptor antagonist. The proportion of β-blockade to α-blockade when given orally is 3:1 and 7:1 when given intravenously. It lowers the blood pressure by blocking α-adrenoceptors in arterioles and thereby reducing the peripheral resistance. Concurrent β-blockade protects the heart from reflex sympathetic drive normally induced by peripheral vasodilatation.

What to use labetalol for
All grades of hypertension, particularly useful when there is tachycardia
Pre-eclampsia

When not to use labetalol
Asthma (worsens)
Cardiogenic shock (further myocardial depression)
Second or third degree heart block

How to use labetalol
- Orally: 100-800 mg 12 hrly
- IV bolus: 10-20 mg over 2 mins, repeat with 40 mg at 10 min intervals as necessary, up to 300 mg in 24 hrs,
  Maximum effect usually occurs within 5 mins and the duration of action is usually 6 hrs
- IV infusion: 20-160 mg/hr
  Available in 20 ml ampoules containing 100 mg labetalol (5 mg/ml).
  Draw up 3 ampoules (60 ml) into a 50 ml syringe
  Rate: 4-32 ml/hr (20-160 mg/hr), adjust rate until satisfactory ↓ BP obtained

How not to use labetalol
Incompatible with sodium bicarbonate

Adverse effects
Postural hypotension
Bradycardia
Heart failure

Cautions
Rare reports of severe hepatocellular damage (usually reversible)
Presence of labetalol metabolites in urine may result in false positive test for phaeochromocytoma.

Organ failure
Hepatic: Reduce dose

NIFEDIPINE

Calcium channel blocker which causes both systemic and coronary vasodilation. By decreasing the afterload it also decreases myocardial oxygen consumption. The onset of action is more rapid after sublingual administration (5 mins compared to 20 mins when given orally).

What to use nifedipine for
Hypertension
Angina

When not to use nifedipine
Congestive heart failure

How to use nifedipine
Orally: 10–40 mg 8 hrly
         Slow-release tablets 30–60 mg once daily
SL: 5–10 mg, repeat every 30–60 mins as necessary

How not to use nifedipine
Do not crush or divide slow-release tablets

Adverse effects
Dizziness
Headache
Hypotension
Heart failure

Cautions
Beta-blockers (increase risk of heart failure and severe hypotension)

Organ failure
Cardiac: Worsens
Renal: Reversible worsening (start with small dose)

NIMODIPINE

A calcium-channel blocker with smooth muscle relaxant effect preferentially in the cerebral arteries. Its use is confined to prevention of vascular spasm after subarachnoid haemorrhage. Nimodipine is used in conjunction with the "triple H" regime of hypertension, hypervolaemia and haemodilution to a haematocrit of 30-33.

What to use nimodipine for
Subarachnoid haemorrhage

What not to use nimodipine for
Hypertension

How to use nimodipine
- IV infusion
  1 mg/hr, ↑ to 2 mg/hr if BP not severely ↓.
  If <70 kg or BP unstable start at 0.5 mg/hr.
  Ready prepared solution - do not dilute.
  But administer into a running infusion (40 ml/hr) of 0.9% saline or 5% dextrose, via a central line.
  Continue for 5-14 days.
  Use only polyethylene or polypropylene infusion sets.
  Protect from light.
- Oral (prophylaxis)
  60 mg every 4 hrs for 21 days

How not to use nimodipine
Avoid PVC infusion sets.
Do not use peripheral venous access.
Do not give nimodipine tablets and IV infusion concurrently.
Avoid concurrent use of other calcium-channel blockers, β-blockers, or nephrotoxic drugs.

Adverse effects
Hypotension (vasodilatation)
Transient ↑ liver enzymes with IV use

Cautions
Hypotension (may be counter-productive by ↓ cerebral perfusion)
Cerebral oedema or severely ↑ ICP
Renal impairment

PHENTOLAMINE

Phentolamine produces peripheral vasodilatation by blocking both α_1 and β_2 adrenergic receptors. Pulmonary vascular resistance and pulmonary arterial pressure are decreased.

What to use phentolamine for
Severe hypertension associated with phaeochromocytoma

When not to use phentolamine
Hypotension

How to use phentolamine
Available in 10 mg ampoules
IV bolus: 2–5 mg, repeat as necessary
IV infusion: 0.1–2 mg/min
Dilute in 0.9% saline or 5% dextrose
Monitor pulse and BP continuously

How not to use phentolamine
Do not use adrenaline, ephedrine, isoprenaline or dobutamine to treat phentolamine-induced hypotension (β_2-effect of these sympathomimetics will predominate causing a further paradoxical $\downarrow$ BP). Treat phentolamine-induced hypotension with noradrenaline.

Adverse effects
Hypotension
Tachycardia and arrhythmias
Dizziness
Nasal congestion

Cautions
Asthma (sulphites in ampoule may lead to hypersensitivity)
IHD

RESPIRATORY DRUGS

CAUSES OF WHEEZING IN THE ICU

- Pre-existing asthma/COAD
- Anaphylactic reaction
- Aspiration pneumonia
- Kinked tracheal tube
- Tracheal tube too far - carinal/bronchial stimulation
- Bronchial secretions
- Pulmonary oedema
- Pneumothorax

SIGNS OF SEVERE ASTHMA NEEDING INTENSIVE CARE

- Tachycardia (HR>130/min)
- Pulsus paradox >20 mmHg
- Tachypnoea (RR>30/min)
- Absent wheezing
- Exhaustion
- Inability to complete a sentence
- $PaCO_2$ normal or increased
- Hypoxia

The selective β_2 agonists such as salbutamol and terbutaline are the treatment of choice for episodes of reversible bronchospasm. Patients with chronic bronchitis and emphysema are often described as having irreversible airways obstruction, but they usually respond partially to the β_2 agonists or to the antimuscarinic drugs ipratropium or oxitropium. There is some evidence that patients who use β_2 agonist on a 'as necessary' basis show greater improvement in their asthma than those using them on a regular basis. In the critically ill these drugs will have to be given either nebulised or intravenously. The tracheobronchial route is preferable because the drug is delivered directly to the bronchioles; smaller doses are then required which causes fewer side-effects. If the bronchospasm is so severe that very little drug gets to the site of action via the tracheobronchial route, then the drug will have to be given IV.

SALBUTAMOL

What to use salbutamol for

Reverse bronchospasm

How to use salbutamol

- Nebuliser: 2.5-5 mg 6 hrly, undiluted (if prolonged delivery time desirable then dilute with 0.9% saline only).
  For patients with chronic bronchitis and hypercapnia, oxygen can be dangerous ($\uparrow$ $PaCO_2$), and nebulisers should be driven by air.
- IV: 5 mg made up to 50 ml with 5% dextrose (100 µg/ml)
  Rate: 200-1200 µg/hr (2-12 ml/hr)

How not to use salbutamol

For nebuliser: Do not dilute in anything other than 0.9% saline (hypotonic solution may cause bronchospasm)

Adverse effects

Tremor
Tachycardia
Paradoxical bronchospasm (stop giving if suspected)
Potentially serious hypokalaemia (potentiated by concomitant treatment with aminophylline, steroids, diuretics and hypoxia)

Cautions

Thyrotoxicosis
In patients already receiving large doses of other sympathomimetic drugs

IPRATROPIUM

An antimuscarinic bronchodilator traditionally regarded as more effective in relieving bronchoconstriction associated with COAD.

What to use ipratropium for
Reverse bronchospasm, particularly in COAD

How to use ipratropium
Nebuliser: 250–500 µg up to 6 hrly, undiluted (if prolonged delivery time desirable then dilute with 0.9% saline only)

For patients with chronic bronchitis and hypercapnia, oxygen can be dangerous ($\uparrow PaCO_2$), and nebulisers should be driven by air.

How not to use ipratropium
For nebuliser: Do not dilute in anything other than 0.9% saline (hypotonic solution may cause bronchospasm)

Adverse effects
Dry mouth
Tachycardia
Paradoxical bronchospasm (stop giving if suspected)
Acute angle closure glaucoma (avoid escape from mask to patient's eyes)

Cautions
Prostatic hypertrophy – urinary retention (unless patient's bladder catheterized)

AMINOPHYLLINE

The ethylenediamine salt of theophylline. It is a non-specific inhibitor of phosphodiesterase, producing increased levels of cAMP. Increased cAMP levels result in:

- Bronchodilation
- CNS stimulation
- Positive inotropic and chronotropic effects
- Diuresis

Theophylline has been claimed to reduce fatigue of diaphragmatic muscles.

What to use aminophylline for
Prevention and treatment of bronchospasm

When not to use aminophylline
Uncontrolled arrhythmias
Hyperthyroidism

How to use aminophylline
Loading dose: 5 mg/kg IV
Dilute in 5% dextrose or 0.9% saline, given over 30 mins, followed by maintenance dose: 0.1-0.8 mg/kg/hr

No loading if already on oral theophylline preparations (toxicity)
Reduce maintenance dose (0.1-0.3 mg/kg/hr) in the elderly and patients with congestive heart failure and liver disease.
Increase maintenance dose (0.8-1 mg/kg/hr) in children (6 months-16 yrs) and young adult smokers.
Monitor plasma level (p 9)

LINE COMPATIBILITY
- Atracurium
- Labetalol
- Morphine
- Pancuronium
- Potassium chloride
- Ranitidine
- Vecuronium

How not to use aminophylline
Rapid IV administration (hypotension, arrhythmias)

Adverse effects
Tachycardia
Arrhythmias
Convulsions

Cautions
Clearance affected by enzyme inducers and inhibitors (p 7)
Concurrent use of erythromycin and ciprofloxacin: Reduce dose

Organ failure
Cardiac: Prolonged half-life (reduce dose)
Hepatic: Prolonged half-life (reduce dose)

DIURETICS
and other drugs working on the kidneys

BUMETANIDE

A potent loop diuretic similar to frusemide. Ototoxicity may be less with bumetanide than with frusemide, but nephrotoxicity may be worse.

What to use bumetanide for
- Acute oliguric renal failure.
- May convert acute oliguric to non-oliguric renal failure. Other measures must be taken to ensure adequate circulating blood volume and renal perfusion pressure.
- Pulmonary oedema
  Secondary to acute left ventricular failure.
- Oedema.
Associated with congestive cardiac failure, hepatic failure and renal disease.

When not to use bumetanide
Oliguria secondary to hypovolaemia

How to use bumetanide
IV bolus: 1-2 mg 1-2 mins, repeat in 2-3 hrs if needed

Adverse effects
Hyponatraemia, hypokalaemia, hypomagnesaemia
Hyperuricaemia, hyperglycaemia
Hypovolaemia
Ototoxicity
Nephrotoxicity
Pancreatitis

Cautions
- Amphotericin (increased risk of hypokalaemia).
- Aminoglycosides (increased nephrotoxicity and ototoxicity).
- Digoxin toxicity (due to hypokalaemia).

Organ failure
Renal: Need to increase dose

DESMOPRESSIN

Pituitary diabetes insipidus (DI) results from a deficiency of antidiuretic hormone (ADH) secretion. Desmopressin is an analogue of ADH. Treatment may be required for a limited period only, in DI following head trauma or pituitary surgery. It is also used in the differential diagnosis of DI. Restoration of the ability to concentrate urine after water deprivation confirms a diagnosis of pituitary DI. Failure to respond occurs in nephrogenic DI.

What to use desmopressin for
Pituitary DI - diagnosis and treatment

How to use desmopressin
* Diagnosis
  Intranasally: 20 µg
  SC/IM: 2 µg
* Treatment
  Intranasally: 10-40 µg daily
  SC/IM/IV: 1-4 µg daily

Monitor fluid intake
Patient should be weighed daily

Adverse effects
Fluid retention
Hyponatraemia
Headache
Nausea and vomiting

Cautions
Renal impairment
Cardiac disease
Hypertension
Cystic fibrosis

FRUSEMIDE

A widely used loop diuretic.

What to use frusemide for

- Acute oliguric renal failure.
- May convert acute oliguric to non-oliguric renal failure. Other measures must be taken to ensure adequate circulaing blood volume and renal perfusion pressure.
- Pulmonary oedema.
  Secondary to acute left ventricular failure.
- Oedema.
  Associated with congestive cardiac failure, hepatic failure and renal disease.

When not to use frusemide

Oliguria secondary to hypovolaemia

How to use frusemide

- IV bolus: 10-40 mg over 3-5 mins
- IV infusion: 2 -10 mg/hr. For high dose parenteral therapy (up to 1000 mg/day)
  Dilute in 250-500 ml of 0.9% saline given at a rate not >240 mg/hr

How not to use frusemide

Dextrose containing fluid is not recommended as a diluent (may precipitate)

Adverse effects

Hyponatraemia, hypokalaemia, hypomagnesaemia
Hyperuricaemia, hyperglycaemia
Ototoxicity
Nephrotoxicity
Pancreatitis

Cautions

Amphotericin (increased risk of hypokalaemia)
Aminoglycosides (increased nephrotoxicity and ototoxicity)
Digoxin toxicity (due to hypokalaemia)

Organ failure

Renal: Need to increase dose

MANNITOL

An alcohol capable of causing an osmotic diuresis. Available as 10% and 20% solutions. Crystallisation may occur at low temperatures. It has a rapid onset of action and duration of action is up to 4 hrs. Rapid infusion of mannitol increases the cardiac output and the BP.

What to use mannitol for

- Cerebral oedema.
- To start a diuresis in oliguric patients.
- To preserve renal function perioperatively in jaundiced patients.
- To initiate diuresis in transplanted kidneys.

When not to use mannitol

Congestive cardiac failure
Pulmonary oedema (acute expansion of blood volume)
Intravascular volume (further ↑ intravascular volume)

How to use mannitol

- Cerebral oedema

IV infusion: 1 g/kg as a 20% solution over 30 mins
100 ml of a 20% solution = 2 g

Weight (kg)	Volume of 20% mannitol at a dose of 1g/kg (ml)
60	300
70	350
80	400
90	450
100	500

- Oliguria

Ensure patient is not hypovolaemic.
IV infusion: 100ml 20% mannitol over 30 mins

- Jaundice

Pre–operative: Insert urinary catheter
500 ml 0.9% saline over 1 hr, 2 hrs before surgery
250 ml 20% mannitol over 30 mins, 1 hr before surgery

Per–operative: 500 ml 20% mannitol if urine output <60 ml/hr
0.9% saline to match urine output

- Kidney transplant

IV infusion: 1 g/kg over 30 mins, given with frusemide 40 mg IV on reperfusion of transplanted kidney.

How not to use mannitol
Do not give in the same line as blood

Adverse effects
Fluid overload
Hyponatraemia and hypokalaemia
Rebound ↑ ICP

Cautions
Extravasation (thrombophlebitis)

Organ failure
Cardiac: Worsens
Renal: Fluid overload

GASTRO-INTESTINAL DRUGS

ANTI-ULCER DRUGS

Critically ill patients are highly stressed and this leads to an increased incidence of peptic ulceration. The risk of stress ulceration is increased in the presence of:

- Sepsis
- Head injury
- Major surgical procedures
- Multiple trauma
- Severe burn injuries
- Respiratory failure
- Severe hepatic failure
- Severe renal failure

Routine use of anti-ulcer drugs to all patients in an ICU is unnecessary. Their use should be restricted to those who have the risk factors described above and should be stopped when patients are established on oral or NG feeding.

RANITIDINE

It is a specific histamine H_2-antagonist which inhibits basal and stimulated secretion of gastric acid, reducing both the volume and the pH of the secretion.

What to use ranitidine for
Peptic ulcer disease
Prophylaxis of stress ulceration
Premedication in patients at risk of acid aspiration

How to use ranitidine
IV bolus: 50 mg 8 hrly
Dilute to 20 ml with 0.9% saline or 5% dextrose and give over 5 mins
In severe renal impairment (CC <10 ml/min): 25 mg 8 hrly

How not to use ranitidine
Do not give rapidly as IV bolus (bradycardia, arrhythmias)

Adverse effects
Hypersensitivity reactions
Bradycardia
Transient and reversible worsening of liver function tests
Reversible leucopaenia and thrombocytopenia

Organ failure
Renal: Reduce dose

SUCRALFATE

A complex of aluminium hydroxide and sulphated sucrose. It acts by protecting the mucosa from acid–pepsin attack.

What to use sucralfate for
Prophylaxis of stress ulceration

What not to use sucralfate for
Severe renal impairment (CC <10 ml/min)

How to use sucralfate
Orally: 1 g suspension 4 hrly

How not to use sucralfate
Do not give ranitidine concurrently (may need acid environment to work)

Adverse effects
Constipation
Diarrhoea

Cautions
Renal impairment

Organ failure
Renal: Aluminium may accumulate

ANTI-EMETICS

- Cyclizine
- Droperidol
- Metoclopramide
- Ondansetron
- Prochlorperazine

TREATMENT OF CONSTIPATION

- Glycerol suppository
- Lactulose

TREATMENT OF DIARRHOEA

- Codeine
- Loperamide

CYCLIZINE

Anti-histamine with antimuscarinic effects.

What to use cyclizine for
Nausea and vomiting.

How to use cyclizine
IM/IV: 50 mg 8 hrly.

Adverse effects
Anticholinergic: drowsiness, dryness of mouth, blurred vision, tachycardia.

Cautions
Sedative effect enhanced by concurrent use of other CNS depressants.

Organ failure
CNS: Sedative effects enhanced.

DROPERIDOL

A butyrophenone with useful anti-emetic properties even at a fraction of the usual neuroleptic dose.

What to use droperidol for
Nausea and vomiting.

When not to use droperidol
Parkinson's disease.

How to use droperidol
IV bolus: 0.625–1.25 mg.
Added to PCAS pumps: 5 mg in 60 mg morphine.

Adverse effects
Drowsiness, apathy, nightmares.
Extrapyramidal movements.

Cautions
Concurrent use of other CNS depressants (enhanced sedation).

Organ failure
CNS: Sedative effects increased.
Hepatic: Can precipitate coma.
Renal: Increased cerebral sensitivity.

METOCLOPRAMIDE

Raises the threshold of the chemoreceptor trigger zone. In high doses it has 5-HT$_3$ antagonist action.

What to use metoclopramide for
Anti-emetic
Promotes gastric emptying
Increases lower oesophageal sphincter tone

How to use metoclopramide
IV/IM: 10 mg 8 hrly

How not to use metoclopramide
Orally not appropriate if actively vomiting
Rapid IV bolus (hypotension)

Adverse effects
Extrapyramidal movements
Neuroleptic malignant syndrome

Cautions
Increased risk of extrapyramidal side-effects occurs in the following:
- Hepatic and renal impairment
- Children, young adults (especially girls) and the very old
- Concurrent use of antipsychotics
- Concurrent use of lithium

Treatment of acute oculogyric crises includes stopping metoclopramide (usually subside within 24 hrs) or giving procyclizine 5-10 mg IV (usually effective within 5 mins).

Organ failure
Hepatic: Reduce dose
Renal: Reduce dose

ONDANSETRON

A specific 5-HT$_3$ antagonist

What to use ondansetron for
Severe post-operative nausea and vomiting
Highly emetogenic chemotherapy

How to use ondansetron
Initial dose: 8 mg slow IV over 15 mins
Followed by continuous IV infusion of 1 mg/hr for up to 24 hr
Dilution: 24 mg ondansetron made up to 48 ml with 0.9% saline or 5% dextrose
Rate of infusion: 2 ml/hr

How not to use ondansetron
Do not give rapidly as IV bolus

Adverse effects
Headaches
Flushing
Constipation
Increases in liver enzymes (transient)

Cautions
Hepatic impairment

Organ failure
Hepatic: Reduced clearance
(moderate or severe liver disease: not >8 mg daily)

PROCHLORPERAZINE

A phenothiazine which inhibits the medullary chemoreceptor trigger zone.

What to use prochlorperazine for
Nausea and vomiting.

When not to use prochlorperazine
Parkinson's disease.

How to use prochlorperazine
IM/IV: 12.5 mg 6 hrly.

Adverse effects
Drowsiness.
Postural hypotension, tachycardia.
Extrapyramidal movements particularly in children, elderly and debilitated.

Cautions
Concurrent use of other CNS depressants (enhanced sedation).

Organ failure
CNS: Sedative effects increased.
Hepatic: Can precipitate coma.
Renal: Increased cerebral sensitivity.

GLYCEROL SUPPOSITORY

Glycerol suppositories act as a rectal stimulant by virtue of the mildly irritant action of glycerol.

What to use glycerol suppository for
Constipation.

When not to use glycerol suppository
Intestinal obstruction.

How to use glycerol suppository
PR: 4 g suppository moistened with water before insertion.

How not to use glycerol suppository
Not for prolonged use.

Adverse effects
Abdominal discomfort.

Cautions
Prolonged use (atonic colon and hypokalaemia).

LACTULOSE

Lactulose is a semi-synthetic disaccharide which is not absorbed from the GI tract. It produces an osmotic diarrhoea of low faecal pH, and discourages the proliferation of ammonia-producing organisms.

What to use lactulose for
Constipation.
Hepatic encephalopathy.

When not to use lactulose
Intestinal obstruction
Galactosaemia

How to use lactulose

- Constipation
  Orally: 15 ml 12 hrly, gradually reduced according to patient's-needs.
  May take up to 48 hrs to act.

- Hepatic encephalopathy
  Orally: 30-50 ml 8 hrly, subsequently adjusted to produce 2-3 soft stools daily.

Adverse effects
Flatulence
Abdominal discomfort

CODEINE PHOSPHATE

Codeine has a low affinity for the μ and κ opioid receptors. It is relatively more effective when given orally than parenterally. It is useful as an anti-tussive and for the treatment of diarrhoea. Side-effects are uncommon and respiratory depression is seldom a problem. This explains its traditional use to provide analgesia for head-injured and neurosurgical patients. Doses above 60 mg do not improve analgesic activity but may increase side-effects. 10% undergoes demethylation to morphine - this possibly contributing to the analgesic effect.

What to use codeine phosphate for
Mild to moderate pain
Diarrhoea and excessive ileostomy output
Antitussive

When not to use codeine phosphate
Airway obstruction

How to use codeine phosphate
Orally: 30-60 mg 4-6 hrly
IM: 30-60 mg 4-6 hrly

How not to use codeine phosphate
Not for IV use

Adverse effects
Drowsiness
Constipation
Nausea and vomiting
Respiratory depression

Cautions
Enhanced sedative and respiratory depression from interaction with:
- Benzodiazepines
- Antidepressants
- Antipsychotics

MAOI (hypertension, hyperpyrexia, convulsions and coma).
Head injury and neurosurgical patients (may exacerbate ↑ ICP as a result of ↑ $PaCO_2$).
May cause renal failure

Organ failure
CNS: Sedative effects increased
Hepatic: Can precipitate coma
Renal: Increased cerebral sensitivity

LOPERAMIDE

Reduces GI motility by direct effect on nerve endings and intramural ganglia within the intestinal wall. Very little is absorbed systemically.

What to use loperamide for
Acute or chronic diarrhoea.

When not to use loperamide
Bowel obstruction.
Toxic megacolon.

How to use loperamide
Orally: 4 mg, then 2 mg after each loose stool to a maximum of 16 mg/day.
Stools should be cultured.

Adverse effects
Bloating
Abdominal pain

ENDOCRINE DRUGS

CORTICOSTEROIDS

While the normal physiological secretion of glucocorticoids from the adrenal cortex is approximately 30 mg cortisol per day, this can increase to 200-400 mg as part of the stress response to major surgery or trauma. Long term therapy can suppress this adrenocortical response to stress. Patients on steroids, or who have taken them within the last 12 months are also at risk of adrenal insufficiency. This may result in life-threatening hypotension, hyponatraemia and hyperkalaemia. The risk is greater when daily oral intake of prednisolone is >7.5 mg.

The aim in synthesising new compounds has been to dissociate glucocorticoid and mineralocorticoid effects.

	Relative potencies		Equivalent dose (mg)
	Glucocorticoid	Mineralcorticoid	
Hydrocortisone	1	1	20
Prednisolone	4	0.25	5
Methylprednisolone	5	⊥	4
Dexamethasone	25	±	0.8
Fludrocortisone	10	300	−

SHORT SYNACTHEN TEST

Prior to starting corticosteroid treatment, it is worth confirming the diagnosis of adrenal insufficiency. Failure of plasma cortisol to rise after IM/IV tetracosactrin 250 μg indicates adrenocortical insufficiency.

Procedure:
> Contact lab first.
> Take blood for cortisol before and 30 mins after IM/IV tetracosactrin 250 μg.

Interpretation:
> A normal response requires an incremental rise of at least 200 nmol/L and a final result must be >500 nmol/L. In the critically ill, values should be much higher. We normally accept a value of 1000 nmol/L anywhere in the test as being sufficient for a septic patient needing ventilatory support

The test is impossible to interpret once hydrocortisone has been started. If urgent treatment is required prior to test, use dexamethasone initially.

DEXAMETHASONE

Dexamethasone has very high glucocorticoid activity and insignificant mineralcorticoid activity, making it particularly suitable for conditions where water retention would be a disadvantage.

What to use dexamethasone for
Cerebral oedema
Laryngeal oedema

How to use dexamethasone
• Cerebral oedema
IV bolus: 8 mg initially, then 4 mg 6 hrly as required for 2–10 days

How not to use dexamethasone
Do not stop abruptly (adrenocortical insufficiency)

Adverse effects
Perineal irritation may follow IV administration of the phosphate ester
Prolonged use may also lead to the following problems:

• Increased susceptibility to infections
• Impaired wound healing
• Peptic ulceration
• Muscle weakness (proximal myopathy)
• Osteoporosis
• Hyperglycaemia

Cautions
Diabetes mellitus
Concurrent use of NSAIDs (increased risk of GI bleeding)

HYDROCORTISONE

Available as the sodium succinate or the phosphate ester.

What to use hydrocortisone for
Adrenal insufficiency (primary or secondary)
Severe bronchospasm
Hypersensitivity reactions (p 18)

What not to use hydrocortisone for
Systemic fungal infections (worsens)

How to use hydrocortisone
Adrenal insufficiency
Major surgery or stress: IV 100–500 mg 6–8 hrly
Minor surgery: IV 50 mg 8–12 hrly
Reduce by 25% per day until normal oral steroids resumed or maintained on 20 mg in the morning and 10 mg in the evening intravenously.

How not to use hydrocortisone
Do not stop abruptly (adrenocortical insufficiency)

Adverse effects
Perineal irritation may follow IV administration of the phosphate ester
Prolonged use may also lead to the following problems:
• Increased susceptibility to infections
• Impaired wound healing
• Peptic ulceration
• Muscle weakness (proximal myopathy)
• Osteoporosis
• Hyperglycaemia

Cautions
Diabetes mellitus

INSULIN

Insulin plays a key role in the regulation of carbohydrate, fat and protein metabolism. Insulin deficiency of resistance may occur in the critically ill patients for several reasons.

What to use insulin for
Hyperglycaemia
Emergency treatment of hyperkalaemia (p 19)

How to use insulin
Soluble insulin (e.g. Actrapid) 50 units made up to 50 ml with 0.9% saline.
Adjust rate according to the sliding scale below.

INSULIN SLIDING SCALE

BM	Rate (ml/hr)
<4	0
4–7	1
7–11	2
11–17	4
>17	6

The energy and carbohydrate intake must be adequate; this may be in the form of entereal or parenteral feeding, or IV infusion of 10% dextrose containing 10-40 mmol/L KCl running at a constant rate appropriate to the patient's fluid requirements (85-125 ml/hr). The blood glucose concentration should be maintained between 4-10 mmol/L.

Monitor: Blood glucose 2 hrly until stable then 4 hrly
          Serum potassium 12 hrly

How not to use insulin
SC administration not recommended for fine control
Adsorption of insulin occurs with PVC bags (use polypropylene syringes)

Adverse effects
Hypoglycaemia

Cautions
Insulin resistance may occur in patients with high levels of IgG antibodies to insulin, obesity, acanthosis nigrans and insulin receptor defects.

HAEMATOLOGICAL AGENTS

APROTININ

Aprotinin is a polypeptide derived from bovine lung. The mechanisms producing the decrease in blood loss are unclear but may be due to its inhibition of plasmin and preservation of platelet membrane binding receptors. There is no risk of developing DVT due to its weak anticoagulant effect.

What to use aprotinin for
- Uncontrolled bleeding caused by hyperplasminaemia.
- Blood conservation - established role in open heart surgery. Some promising reports of their use in orthopaedic procedures, in the critically ill and after liver tranplantation.

How to use aprotinin
- Uncontrolled bleeding due to hyperplasminaemia (not correctable by blood products)

  Loading dose of 50 ml (500 000 units) to 100 ml (1 million units) given by slow IV infusion over 20-30 mins The initial 5 ml (50 000 units) should be given slowly, over 5 mins, (to detect allergy).

  If necessary, further 20 ml (200 000 units) every hour may be given until bleeding stops

- Blood conservation.

  Loading dose of 200 ml (2 million units) given by slow IV infusion over 30-60 mins. The initial 5 ml (50 000 units) should be given slowly, over 5 mins (to detect allergy)

  If necessary, further 50ml (500 000 units) every hour may be given.

Adverse effects
Generally well tolerated
Thrombophlebitis
Hypersensitivity

Cautions
Incompatible in lines containing corticosteroids, heparin, nutrient solutions containing amino acids or fat emulsions, and tetracyclines.

CYCLOSPORIN A

Cyclosporin is a cyclic peptide molecule derived from a soil fungus. It is a potent nephrotoxin, producing interstitial renal fibrosis with tubular atrophy. Monitoring of cyclosporin blood level is essential.
Normal range: 100–300 µg/L
For renal transplants: lower end of range
For heart/lung/liver: upper end of range

What to use cyclosporin for
Prevention of organ rejection after transplantation

How to use cyclosporin
- IV dose: 1–5 mg/kg/day

To be diluted 1 in 20 to 1 in 100 with 0.9% saline or 5% dextrose
To be given over 2–6 hrs
Infusion should be completed within 12 hrs if using PVC lines
Switch to oral for long term therapy
- Oral dose: 1.5 times IV dose given 12 hrly

Monitor: Hepatic function
       Renal function
       Cyclosporin blood level (pre-dose sample)

How not to use cyclosporin
Must not be given as IV bolus.
Do not infuse at a rate >12 hrs if using PVC lines – leaching of phthalates from the PVC.

Adverse effects
Enhanced renal sensitivity to insults
↑ Plasma urea and serum creatinine secondary to glomerulosclerosis
Hypertension – responds to conventional antihypertensives
Hepatocellular damage (↑ transaminases)
Hyperuricaemia
Gingival hypertrophy
Hirsuitism
Tremors or seizures at high serum levels

Cautions
↑ susceptibility to infections and lymphoma
↑ nephrotoxic effects with concurrent use of other nephrotoxic drugs

ERYTHROPOEITIN

Epoetin (recombinant human erythropoetin) is available as epoetin alpha and beta. Both are similar in clinical efficacy and can be used interchangeably.

What to use erythropoeitin for
- Anaemia associated with erythropoetin deficiency in chronic renal failure
- Severe anaemia caused by blood loss in Jehovah's witness

What not to use erythropoeitin for
Uncontrolled hypertension
Anaemia due to iron, folic acid or vitamin B_{12} deficiency

How to use erythropoeitin
- Chronic renal failure

Aim to increase haemoglobin concentration at rate not >2 g/100 ml per month to stable level of 10-12 g/100 ml.
SC (max. 1 ml per injection site) or IV over 2 mins
Initially 50 units/kg 3 times weekly increased according to response in steps of 25 units/kg at intervals of 4 weeks.
Maintenance dose (when haemoglobin 10-12 g/100ml) 50-300 units/kg weekly in 2-3 divided doses.

- Severe anaemia due to blood loss in Jehovah's witness

150-300 units/kg daily SC until desired haemoglobin reached.
Supplementary iron (e.g. ferrous sulphate 200 mg PO) and O_2 is mandatory.

Monitor: BP (↑ BP)
               FBC (↑ haemoglobin, ↑ platelet)
               U&Es (↑ urea, ↑ creatinine, ↑ phosphate)
               Serum ferritin

How not to use erythropoeitin
Avoid contact of reconstituted injection with glass; use only plastic materials

Adverse effects
Dose–dependent increase in BP and platelet count
Flu-like symptoms (reduced if IV given over 5 mins)
Shunt thrombosis
Hyperkalaemia
Increase in plasma urea, creatinine and phosphate
Convulsions
Skin reactions
Palpebral oedema
Myocardial infarction
Anaphylaxis

Cautions

Hypertension (stop if uncontrolled)
Ischaemic vascular disease
Thrombocytosis (monitor platelet count for first 8 weeks)
Epilepsy
Malignant disease
Chronic liver disease

HEPARIN

What to use heparin for
- Prophylaxis of DVT and PE
- Treatment of DVT and PE
- Extracorporeal circuits

What not to use heparin for
Haemophilia and other haemorrhagic disorders
Peptic ulcer
Cerebral haemorrhage
Severe hypertension
Severe liver disease (including oesophageal varices)
Severe renal failure
Thrombocytopenia
Hypersensitivity to heparin

How to use heparin
- Prophylaxis of DVT and PE
  SC: 5000 units 8-12 hrly until patient is ambulant.
- Treatment of DVT and PE
  IV: Loading dose of 5000 units followed by continuous infusion of 1000-2000 units/hr.
  24 000 units heparin made up to 48 ml with 0.9% saline (5000 units/ml). Check APTT 6 hrs after loading dose and adjust rate to keep APTT 1.5-2.5 times normal.
  Start oral warfarin as soon as possible
- Haemofiltration.

Adverse effects
Haemorrhage
Skin necrosis
Thrombocytopenia
Hypersensitivity
Osteoporosis after prolonged use

Cautions
Hepatic and renal impairment (avoid if severe)

PROSTACYCLIN

It has a half-life of only 3 mins and must be given by continuous IV infusion. It is a potent vasodilator and therefore its side-effects include flushing, headaches, and hypotension. It is used when heparin is contraindicated in renal dialysis to inhibit platelet aggregation.

What to use prostacyclin for
- Haemofiltration
- ARDS

How to use prostacyclin
Available in vials containing 500 μg epoprostenol. Store in fridge.
Reconstitute the powder with the 50 ml diluent provided (concentration 10,000 nanogram/ml).
Further dilute this 50 ml concentrate in 200 ml 0.9 % saline i.e. 250 ml bag with 50 ml discarded (concentration 2000 nanogram/ml).
IV infusion: 2-5 nanogram/kg/min

Dosage chart: ml/hr

Weight: kg	Dose: nanogram/kg/min			
	2	3	4	5
50	3	4.5	6	7.5
60	3.6	5.4	7.2	9
70	4.2	6.3	8.4	10.5
80	4.8	7.2	9.6	12
90	5.4	8.1	10.8	13.5
100	6	9	12	15

Adverse effects
Flushing
Headaches
Hypotension
Bradycardia

Cautions
Epoprostenol may potentiate heparin

PROTAMINE

Available as a 1% (10 mg/ml) solution of protamine sulphate. Although it is used to neutralise the anticoagulant action of heparin, if used in excess it has anticoagulant effect.

What to use protamine for
Neutralise the anticoagulant action of heparin

How to use protamine
1 ml of 1% (10 mg) protamine is required to neutralise 1000 units of heparin given in the previous 15 mins.
As more time elapses after the heparin injection, proportionally less protamine is required.
Slow IV injection 5 ml 1% over 10 mins
Ideally, the dosage should be guided by serial measurements of APTT/ACT and the rate guided by watching the direct arterial BP.

How not to use protamine
Rapid IV bolus

Adverse effects
Hypersensitivity
Rapid IV administration – pulmonary vasoconstriction, ↓ left atrial pressure and hypotension.

Cautions
Hypersensitivity (severe hypotension may respond to fluid loading)

TRANEXAMIC ACID

Tranexamic acid is another antifibrinolytic employed in blood conservation. It acts by inhibiting plasminogen activation.

What to use tranexamic acid for

- Uncontrolled haemorrhage following prostatectomy or dental extraction in haemophiliacs
- Thrombolytic therapy overdose
- Haemorrhage when fibrinolysis is presented or suspected.

When not to use tranexamic acid

Thromboembolic disease

How to use tranexamic acid

Orally: 1–1.5 g 6–12 hrly
IV: 0.5–1 g   8 hrly, given over 3–5 mins

How not to use tranexamic acid

Rapid IV bolus

Adverse effects

Giddiness on rapid IV injection

Cautions

Renal impairment (reduce dose)

ELECTROLYTES AND VITAMINS

MAGNESIUM

Hypomagnesaemia may result from failure to supply adequate intake, from excess NG drainage or suctioning, or in acute pancreatitis. It is usually accompanied by a loss of potassium. The patient may become confused, irritable with muscle twitching.

Normal range: 0.7-1.0 mmol/L

What to use magnesium sulphate for

Hypomagnesaemia

What not to use magnesium sulphate for

Hypocalcaemia
Hypermagnesaemia
Heart block
Oliguria

How to use magnesium sulphate

Magnesium sulphate solution for injection
1 g = 8 mEq = 4 mmol

Concentration %	g/ml	mEq/ml	mmol/ml
10	0.1	0.8	0.4
25	0.25	2	1
50	0.5	4	2

IV infusion: 10 mmol magnesium sulphate made up to 50 ml with 5% dextrose
Do not give at a rate >30 mmol/hr
Repeat until plasma level is normal
Concentrations <20% are suitable for peripheral IV administration
Monitor: BP, respiratory rate
ECG
Tendon reflexes
Renal function
Serum magnesium level
Maintain urine output >30 ml/hr

How not to use magnesium sulphate
Rapid IV infusion can cause respiratory or cardiac arrest

Adverse effects
Respiratory depression
Bradycardia, arrhythmias and hypotension
Muscle weakness and paralysis

Cautions
Renal impairment – reduce dose

Organ failure
Renal: Slower infusion rate and closer monitoring for signs of
toxicity

PHOSPHATES

Hypophosphataemia may lead to muscle weakness and is a cause of difficulty in weaning a patient from mechanical ventilation. Causes of hypophosphataemia in the critically ill include failure of supplementation e.g. during TPN, use of insulin and high concentration glucose, use of loop diuretics and low dose dopamine.
Normal range: 0.8-1.4 mmol/L

What to use phosphate for
Hypophosphataemia

When not to use phosphate
Hypocalcaemia (further $\downarrow Ca^{2+}$)

How to use phosphate
Available in ampoules of:
Potassium hydrogen phosphate 5 ml 17.42% (potassium 2 mmol/ml, phosphate 1 mmol/ml)
Sodium hydrogen phosphate 10 ml 17.91% (sodium 1 mmol/ml, phosphate 0.5 mmol/ml)
IV infusion: 10 mmol phosphate (K/Na) made up to 50 ml with 5% dextrose or 0.9% saline, given over 12 hrs
Do not give at a rate >10 mmol over 12 hrs
Repeat until plasma level is normal
Monitor serum calcium, phosphate, potassium, and sodium daily

How not to use phosphate
Do not give rapidly

Adverse effects
Hypocalcaemia, hypomagnesaemia, hyperkalaemia, hypernatraemia
Arrhythmias, hypotension
Ectopic calcification

Cautions
Renal impairment
Concurrent use of potassium-sparing diuretics or ACE-I with potassium phosphate may result in hyperkalaemia
Concurrent use of corticosteroids with sodium phosphate may result in hypernatraemia

Organ failure
Renal: Risk of hyperphosphataemia

POTASSIUM

What to use potassium for
Hypokalaemia

When not to use potassium
Severe renal failure
Severe tissue trauma
Untreated Addison's disease

How to use potassium
Potassium chloride 1.5 g (20 mmol K^+) in 10 ml ampoules
Dilute in 5% dextrose or 0.9% saline and make up to 50 ml
Do not give at a rate >20 mmol/hr
Monitor serum potassium regularly
Check serum magnesium in refractory hypokalaemia

LINE COMPATIBILITY
- Adrenaline
- Aminophylline
- Digoxin
- Dobutamine
- Dopamine
- Fentanyl
- Frusemide
- Heparin
- Insulin
- Magnesium sulphate
- Morphine
- Noradrenaline
- Sodium bicarbonate

How not to use potassium
Avoid extravasation and do not give IM or SC (severe pain and tissue necrosis)

Adverse effects
Muscle weakness
Arrhythmias

Cautions
Renal impairment
Concurrent use of potassium-sparing diuretics or ACE-I
Hypokalaemia is frequently associated with hypomanesaemia.

Organ failure
Renal: Risk of hyperkalaemia

ZINC

Zinc deficiency can occur in patients on inadequate diets, in malabsorption, with increased catabolism due to trauma, burns and protein-losing conditions, and during prolonged TPN.
Hypoproteinaemia spuriously lowers plasma zinc levels.
Normal range: 12-23 µmol/L

What to use zinc for
Zinc deficiency

How to use zinc
Oral: Zinc sulphate effervescent tablet 200 mg 1-3 times daily after food

Adverse effects
Abdominal pains
Dyspepsia

BONE MARROW RESCUE FOLLOWING NITROUS OXIDE

- Folinic acid 15 mg IV for 2 days
- Vitamin B12 1 mg IV for 2 days

The use of nitrous oxide for anaesthesia in excess of 2 hrs inactivates vitamin B12 and may lead to impaired DNA synthesis and megaloblastic bone marrow haemopoiesis. In fit patients this is of little significance, but in the critically ill it may increase mortality. Haemopoeitic changes induced by nitrous oxide can be reversed by folinic acid. Vitamin B12 is given to replace that which has been inactivated. Both should be given to critically ill patients following surgery in which nitrous oxide was used as part of the anaesthetic for >2 hrs.

VITAMIN K

Vitamin K is necessary for the production of prothrombin, factors VII, IX and X. It is found primarily in leafy green vegetables and is additionally synthesised by bacteria that colonise the gut. Because it is fat-soluble, it requires bile salts for absorption from the gut. Patients with biliary obstruction or hepatic disease may become deficient. Vitamin K deficiency frequently occurs in hospitalised patients because of poor diet, parenteral nutrition, recent surgery, antibiotic therapy, and uraemia.

What to use vitamin K for
Liver disease
Reversal of warfarin

What not to use vitamin K for
Reversal of warfarin when good control of INR required (use FFP)

How to use vitamin K
Dose: 1–10 mg IV bolus given over 3–5 mins
Maximum 40 mg in 24 hrs
Monitor INR

How not to use vitamin K
Do not give IM injections in patients with abnormal clotting (intramuscular haemorrhages/abscesses)

Adverse effects
Hypersensitivity (if dissolved in cremaphor)

Cautions
Onset of action slow (use FFP if rapid effect needed)

ANTI-MICROBIAL DRUGS

A close liaison with the microbiologists is important for the correct usage of these drugs and to prevent emergence of resistant strains. They may either be used prophylactically post-operatively or used for treating established infection based on culture results. Before a positive culture, the best guess antimicrobial therapy may be chosen for a clinically septic patient. The choice of agent(s) is dependent on a knowledge of the organisms likely to be involved. It is essential to obtain appropriate specimens for microbiological examination, before starting 'blind' therapy. It is also good practice to have stop or review dates to avoid unnecessarily prolonged treatment or side effects.

Although the majority of antibiotics are relatively safe drugs, important toxic effects do occur, particularly in the presence of other disease states. In addition, antibiotics may result in secondary yeast or fungal infection, or may facilitate the growth of *Clostridium difficile*, a cause of pseudomembranous colitis.

Infection is not the only cause of pyrexia. It is worth bearing in mind the phenomenon of antibiotic fever which results in a pyrexia in the absence of an infection, the fever subsiding when the antibiotic is stopped.

NON-INFECTIVE CAUSES OF PYREXIA

- **Cancer**
  Lymphoma
  Leukaemia
  Hypernephroma
  Hepatoma
  Pancreatic carcinoma
- **Connective tissue disease**
  Systemic lupus erythematosus
  Polyarteritis nodosa
  Polymyalgia/cranial arteritis
- **Drugs**
  Antibiotics
- **Sarcoidosis**
- **Rheumatoid disease**
- **Blood/blood product transfusion**
- **Malignant hyperpyrexia**

BACTERIAL GRAM STAINING

	Positive	Negative
COCCI	Enterococci Pneumococcus Staphylococcus Streptococcus	Moraxella catarrhalis Neisseria
RODS	Actinomyces Clostridium Corynebacterium	Bacteroides Escherichia coli Haemophilus influenzae Klebsiella Legionella Proteus Pseudomonas Salmonellae Serratia Shigellae

ANTIBIOTICS: SENSITIVITIES

Antibiotic columns (left to right): Ampicillin, Benzylpenicillin, Cefuroxime, Cefotaxime, Ceftazidime, Ciprofloxacin, Erythromycin, Flucloxacillin, Gentamicin, Imipenem, Meropenem, Metronidazole, Vancomycin

Organism rows:
- S. aureus
- MRSA
- S. pyogenes
- S. pneumoniae
- E. faecalis
- H. influenzae
- E. coli
- Klebsiella spp
- N. meningitidis
- P. mirabilis
- Serratia spp
- Ps. aeruginosa
- B. fragilis
- Other anaerobes

Legend: ■ Sensitive   ▨ Some strains resistant   □ Resistant

When referring to this chart it is important to bear in mind the following:

- There is increasing antibiotics resistance in many organisms.
- There may be a great difference between antibiotic sensitivity determined in-vitro and clinical use.
- There are great geographical variations in antibiotic sensitivity, not only between different countries, but also between different hospitals.
- Flucloxacillin may have activity against *S. pneumoniae,* it is not used to treat a pneumococcal pneumonia.
- *N. meningitidis* is not resistant to imipenem, but it would not be used for treatment beacause of neurotoxicity.
- *N. meningitidis* is not resistant to cefuroxime, although it would not be used for treatment of meningitis beacause of a high relapse rate.

AMPICILLIN

Ampicillin is active against Gram −ve rods such as S*almonella, Shigella, E.coli, H.influenzae* and *Proteus*. It is ineffective against *Pseudomonas, Klebsiella* and penicillinase-producing *S. aureus* and *E. coli*. Almost all staphylococci, 50% *E. coli* and 15% *H. influenzae* are now resistant. Amoxycillin is similar but better absorbed orally.

What to use ampicillin for
Urinary tract infections
Respiratory tract infections

How to use ampicillin
IV: 0.5-1 g diluted in 10 ml WFI, 4-6 hrly over 3-4 mins

In renal impairment:

How not to use ampicillin
Not for intrathecal use (encephalopathy)
Do not mix in the same syringe with an aminoglycoside (efficacy of aminoglycoside reduced).

CC (ml/min)	Dose (g)	Interval (hr)
10-20	0.5-1	8
<10	0.5-1	12

Adverse effects
Hypersensitivity
Skin rash increases in patients with infectious mononucleosis (90%), chronic lymphocytic leukaemia and HIV infections (stop drug).

Cautions
Severe renal impairment (reduce dose, rashes more common)
Penicillin hypersensitivity

BENZYLPENICILLIN

Benzylpenicillin can only be given parenterally and is susceptible to penicillinase-producing *S.aureus*.

What to use benzylpenicillin for
Infective endocarditis
Most streptococcal and pneumococcal infections
Gas gangrene and prophylaxis in limb amputation
Pneumococcal and meningococcal meningitis
Tetanus

How to use benzylpenicillin
IV: 600-1200 mg diluted in 10 ml WFI, 6 hrly over 3-4 mins
Max. 7.2 g/24 hrs for infective endocarditis
Max. 14.4 g/24 hrs for pneumococcal and meningococcal meningitis
Give at a rate not >300 mg/min
In severe renal impairment (CC<10 ml/min): Max. 6 g/24 hrs

How not to use benzylpenicillin
Not for intrathecal use (encephalopathy)
Do not mix in the same syringe with an aminoglycoside (efficacy of aminoglycoside reduced).

Adverse effects
Hypersensitivity
Haemolytic anaemia
Transient neutropenia and thrombocytopenia
Convulsions (high dose or renal failure)

Cautions
Anaphylactic reactions frequent (1:100,000)
Severe renal impairment (reduce dose, high doses may cause convulsions)

CEPHALOSPORINS

Their major advantages over the penicillins are that they are resistant to penicillinase-producing *S.aureus* and have a broader range of activity. Like penicillins, they inhibit cell wall synthesis. Their broad spectrum of activity is useful when the precise nature of the infection is unknown, but their indiscriminate use may encourage superinfection with resistant bacteria or fungi.

CEFOTAXIME

A third generation cephalosporin whose activity against Gram +ve organisms, most notably *S. aureus* is diminished in comparison to second generation cephalosporins, while action against Gram − ve organisms is enhanced.

What to use cefotaxime for
Surgical prophylaxis
Haemophilus epiglottitis
Meningitis
Peritonitis
Pneumonia
Urinary tract infections

What not to use cefotaxime for
Hypersensitivity to cephalosporins
Serious penicillin hypersensitivity (10% cross–sensitivity)
Porphyria

How to use cefotaxime
IV: 2-6 g daily in divided dose depending on severity of infection
Dilute in 5 ml WFI, given IV over 3-5 mins

Infection	Dose (g)	Interval (hr)
Mild–moderate	1	12
Moderate–serious	1	8
Life threatening	2	8

In severe renal impairment (CC<10 ml/min): half dose

Adverse effects
Hypersensitivity
Transient ↑ LFTs
Pseudomembranous colitis (more likely with high doses)

Cautions
Concurrent use of nephrotoxic drugs (aminoglycosides, loop diuretics)
Severe renal impairment (half dose)
False + ve urinary glucose (if tested for reducing substances)
False + ve Coombs' test

CEFTAZIDIME

A third generation cephalosporin whose activity against Gram +ve organisms, most notably *S. aureus* is diminished in comparison to second generation cephalosporins, while action against Gram −ve organisms is enhanced.

What to use ceftazidime for
Surgical prophylaxis
Haemophilus epiglottitis
Peritonitis
Pneumonia
Urinary tract infections

What not to use ceftazidime for
Hypersensitivity to cephalosporins
Serious penicillin hypersensitivity (10% cross-sensitivity)
Porphyria
Meningitis

How to use ceftazidime
IV: 0.5-2 g 8-12 hrly depending on severity of infection
Dilute in 5 ml WFI, given over 3-5 mins

Infection	Dose (g)	Interval (hr)
Mild–moderate	0.5 – 1	12
Moderate–serious	1	8
Life threatening	2	8

In renal impairment:

CC (ml/min)	Dose (g)	Interval (hr)
20–50	1	8 – 12
10–20	1	12 – 24
<10	0.5	24 – 48

Adverse effects
Hypersensitivity
Transient (liver function tests)
Pseudomembranous colitis (more likely with high doses)

Cautions
Renal impairment (reduce dose)
Concurrent use of nephrotoxic drugs (aminoglycosides, loop diuretics)
False −ve urinary glucose (if tested for reducing substances)
False +ve Coombs' test

CEFUROXIME

A second generation cephalosporin widely used in combination with metronidazole in the post-operative period following most abdominal procedures. Has greater activity against *S. aureus* (including penicillinase-producing) and *H. influenzae* compared with the third generation cephalosporins, but not active against MRSA, *Enterococcus* and *Ps. aeruginosa.*

What to use cefuroxime for
Surgical prophylaxis
Haemophilus epiglottitis
Peritonitis
Pneumonia
Urinary tract infections

What not to use cefuroxime for
Hypersensitivity to cephalosporins
Serious penicillin hypersensitivity (10% cross-sensitivity)
Porphyria
Meningitis

How to use cefuroxime
IV: 0.75-1.5 g 6-8 hrly
Dilute with 20 ml WFI, given over 3-5 mins

CC (ml/min)	Dose (g)	Interval (hr)
10 – 20	0.75	6 – 8
<10	0.75	8 – 12

In renal impairment:

Adverse effects
Hypersensitivity
Transient ↑ LFTs
Pseudomembranous colitis (more likely with high doses)

Cautions
Hypersensitivity to penicillins
Renal impairment

CO-TRIMOXAZOLE

Sulphamethoxazole and trimethoprim are used in combination because of their synergistic activity. Increasing resistance to sulphonamides and the high incidence of sulphonamide-related side-effects have diminished the value of co-trimoxazole. Trimethoprim alone is now preferred for urinary tract infections and exacerbations of chronic bronchitis. However, high dose co-trimoxazole is the preferred treatment for *Pneumocystis carinii* pneumonia (PCP). It has certain theoretical advantages over pentamidine: pentamidine accumulates slowly in the lung parenchyma and improvement may occur more slowly, co-trimoxazole has a broad spectrum of activity and may treat any bacterial co-pathogens.

What to use co-trimoxazole for
Severe PCP

What not to use co-trimoxazole for
Pregnancy
Severe renal/hepatic failure
Blood disorders
Porphyria

How to use co-trimoxazole
• Severe PCP
60 mg/kg 12 hrly IV for 14 days followed orally for a further 7 days
IV infusion. Dilute every 1 ml (96 mg) in 25 ml 5% dextrose or 0.9% saline, given over 1.5-2 hrs. If fluid restriction necessary, dilute in half the amount of 5% dextrose.

Adjuvant corticosteroid (methylprednisolone 1 g daily for 3 days) given early improves survival.

In renal impairment (CC <20 ml/min): reduce dose to 75%

Note:
• Treatment should be stopped if rashes or serious blood disorders develop.
• A decrease in white cell count should be treated with folinic acid and a dose reduction to 75%.
• AZT (Zidovudine) must be stopped while giving high dose co-trimoxazole as the combination is likely to produce a decrease in white cell count.

How not to use co-trimoxazole

Concurrent use of both co-trimoxazole and pentamidine is not of benefit and may increase the incidence of serious side-effects.

Adverse effects

Nausea, vomiting and diarrhoea
    (including pseudomembranous colitis).

Rashes (including Stevens-Johnson syndrome).

Blood disorders
    (includes leucopenia, thrombocytopaenia, anaemia).

Fluid overload (due to large volumes required).

Cautions

Renal impairment (rashes and blood disorders increase, may cause further deterioration in renal function).
Elderly

ERYTHROMYCIN

It has an antibacterial spectrum similar, but not identical, to that of penicillin; it is thus an alternative in penicillin-allergic patients.

What to use erythromycin for
Alternative to penicillin
Pneumonia, particularly caused by atypical organisms
Legionnaire's disease

How to use erythromycin
IV infusion: 0.5–1 g 6 hrly
Reconstitute in 20 ml WFI, then dilute 250 ml 0.9% saline, given over 1 hr.
If fluid retriction necessary, dissolve in 50 ml 5% dextrose and given into a central vein over 1 hr.

In severe renal impairment: Max. 1.5g daily

How not to use erythromycin
IV bolus
Do not use concurrently with astemizole or terfenadine (arrhythmias).

Adverse effects
Hypersentivity reactions
Reversible hearing loss with large doses
Cholestatic jaundice if given >14 days
Prolongation of QT interval

Cautions
↑ Plasma levels of alfentanil, midazolam and theophylline (enzyme inhibition)
Severe renal impairment (ototoxicity)
Hepatic disease

FLUCLOXACILLIN

What to use flucloxacillin for

Infections caused by penicillinase-producing staphylococci:

- Cellulitis
- Endocarditis
- Adjunct in pneumonia

When not to use flucloxacillin

Penicillin hypersensitivity

How to use flucloxacillin

IV: 0.5-1 g every 6 hrs
Reconstitute in 10 ml WFI, given over 3-5 mins
For severe infections double the dose

How not to use flucloxacillin

Not for intrathecal use (encephalopathy)
Do not mix in the same syringe with an aminoglycoside (efficacy of aminoglycoside reduced).

Adverse effects

Hypersensitivity
Haemolytic anaemia
Transient neutropenia and thrombocytopenia
Cholestatic jaundice
 – ↑ risk with treatment >2 weeks and increasing age
 – may occur up to several weeks after stopping treatment

GENTAMICIN

This is the aminoglycoside of choice in the UK. It is inactive against anaerobes and has poor activity against haemolytic streptococci and pneumococci. When used for the 'blind' therapy of undiagnosed serious infections it is usually given with a penicillin and/or metronidazole. It is not appreciably absorbed orally and is excreted unchanged by the kidneys. In renal impairment the half-life is prolonged.

Most side-effects are related to sustained high trough concentrations. Efficacy, on the other hand, is related to peak concentrations that are well in excess of the minimum inhibitory concentration of the infecting organism.

What to use gentamicin for
Septicaemia (with a penicillin and/or metronidazole)
Endocarditis (with a penicillin)
Hospital acquired pneumonia
Severe pseudomonal infections (with piperacillin)
Enterococcal infections (with a penicillin and/or metronidazole)

When not to use gentamicin
Pregnancy
Myasthenia gravis

How to use gentamicin
IV: 1.5 mg/kg IV 8 hrly, given over 3-5 mins

CC (ml/min)	Dose (mg/kg)	Interval (hr)
20 – 50	1.5	12 – 24
10 – 20	1 – 1.5	12 – 24
<10	1	24 – 48

In renal impairment:
Monitor plasma level (p 9): adjust dose/interval accordingly
Recent meta-analysis shows that single daily doses of aminoglycosides (4.5 -6 mg/kg) were about 25% less nephrotoxic and as effective as multiple daily doses.

How not to use gentamicin
Do not mix in a syringe with penicillins (aminoglycosides inactivated)

Adverse effects

- Nephrotoxicity
  ↑ risk with amphotericin, bumetanide, frusemide
- Ototoxicity
  ↑ risk with pre-existing renal insufficiency, elderly, bumetanide, frusemide
- Prolonged neuromuscular blockade
  May be clinically significant in patients being weaned from mechanical ventilation

Cautions

Renal impairment (reduce dose)
Concurrent use of:

- Amphotericin –↑ nephrotoxicity
- Bumetanide, frusemide – ↑ ototoxicity
- Neuromuscular blockers – prolonged muscle weakness

Organ failure

Renal: Increased plasma concentration. ↑ ototoxicity and nephro-toxicity.

IMIPENEM AND CILASTIN

Imipenem is given in combination with cilastin, a specific inhibitor of the renal enzyme dehydopeptidase-1 that inactivates imipenem. Imipenem has an extremely wide spectrum of activity, including most aerobic and anaerobic Gram – ve and Gram + ve bacteria.

What to use imipenem for
Mixed aerobic/anaerobic infections
Surgical prophylaxis

What not to use imipenem for
CNS infections (neurotoxicity)
Meningitis (neurotoxicity)

How to use imipenem
IV infusion: 0.5-1 g 6-8 hrly depending on severity of infection.

Dilute with 0.9% saline or 5% dextrose to a concentration of 5 mg/ml.

> 500 mg: add 100 ml diluent, infuse over 30 mins
> 1 g: add 200 ml diluent, infuse over 60 mins

In renal impairment:

CC (ml/min)	Dose (g)	Interval (hr)
20 – 50	0.5	6 – 8
10 – 20	0.5	8 – 12
‹10	0.3	12 – 24

How not to use imipenem
Not compatible with diluents containing lactate

Adverse effects
Hypersensitivity reactions
Blood disorders
Positive Coombs' test
↑ Liver function tests, serum creatinine and blood urea
Myoclonic activity
Convulsions (high doses or renal impairment)

Cautions
Hypersensitivity to penicillins and cephalosporins
Renal impairment (reduce dose)
Elderly

MEROPENEM

Meropenem is similar to imipenem but is stable to the renal enzyme dehydopeptidase-1 which inactivates imipenem. Meropenem has an extremely wide spectrum of activity, including most aerobic and anaerobic Gram – ve and Gram + ve bacteria.

What to use meropenem for
Pneumonias
Peritonitis
Septicaemia
Meningitis
Infections in neutropenic patients
Chronic lower respiratory tract infections in cystic fibrosis patients

What not to use meropenem for
Hypersensitivity to meropenem
Infections caused by MRSA and *E. faecium*

How to use meropenem
IV bolus: 0.5-1 g 8 hrly, given over 5 mins, or IV infusion over 15-30 mins
But for meningitis, increase to 2 g 8 hrly; for cystic fibrosis, up to 2 g 8 hrly

In renal impairment:

CC (ml/min)	Dose*	Interval (hr)
26 – 50	one unit dose	12
10 – 25	½ unit dose	12
<10	½ unit dose	24

*based on unit doses of 0.5g ,1g, 2g

Meropenem is cleared by haemodialysis – give at completion of haemodiaysis

Adverse effects
Thrombophlebitis
Hypersensitivity reactions
Positive Coombs' test
Reversible thrombocythaemia, thrombocytopenia, eosinophilia and neutropenia
Abnormal LFTs ($\uparrow$ bilirubin, transaminases and alkaline phosphatase)
Convulsions (less risk than imipenem/cilastin)

Cautions
Hypersensitivity to penicillins and cephalosporins
Hepatic impairment (monitor LFTs)
Concurrent use of nephrotoxic drugs

Organ failure
Hepatic: May worsen LFTs
Renal: Reduce dose

METRONIDAZOLE

High activity against anaerobic bacteria and protozoa. It is the drug of choice for antibiotic -associated pseudomembranous colitis.

What to use metronidazole for
Pseudomembranous colitis
Anaerobic infections
Protozoal infections

How to use metronidazole
- Pseudomembranous colitis
Orally: 400 mg 8 hrly
- Anaerobic infections
IV: 500 mg 8 hrly
PR: 1 g 8 hrly

Adverse effects
Nausea and vomiting
Unpleasant taste
Rashes, urticaria and angioedema
Peripheral neuropathy (prolonged treatment)

Cautions
Hepatic impairment
Disulfiram-like reaction with alcohol

PENTAMIDINE

What to use pentamidine for
Alternative treatment for severe PCP

How to use pentamidine
IV: 4 mg/kg every 24 hrs for at least 14 days
Dilute in 250 ml 5% dextrose, given over 1-2 hrs

In renal impairment:

CC (ml/min)	Dose (mg/kg)	Interval (hr)
10 –50	4	36
<10	4	48

Adjuvant corticosteroid (methylprednisolone 1 g daily for 3 days) given early improves survival.

How not to use pentamidine
Nebulised route not recommended in severe PCP ($\downarrow$ PaO$_2$)
Concurrent use of both co-trimoxazole and pentamidine is not of benefit and may increase the incidence of serious side-effects.

Adverse effects
Acute renal failure (usually isolated $\uparrow$ serum creatinine)
Leucopenia, thrombocytopenia
Severe hypotension
Hypoglycaemia
Pancreatitis
Arrhythmias

Cautions
Blood disorders
Hypotension
Renal/hepatic impairment

PIPERACILLIN

One of the antipseudomonal penicillins indicated for treatment of serious infections caused by *Ps. aeruginosa* although they also have activity against other Gram –ve bacilli including *Proteus* spp. and *B. fragilis*. Tazocin® (piperacillin with the beta–lactamase inhibitor tazobactam) is active against beta–lactamase producing bacteria resistant to piperacillin. For pseudomonas septicaemia piperacillin should be given with an aminoglycoside e.g. gentamicin as there is a synergistic effect.

What to use piperacillin for
Infections due to *Ps. aeruginosa*

What not to use piperacillin for
Penicillin hypersensitivity

How to use piperacillin
8–24 g daily in divided doses depending on severity of infection
Dilute in 50 ml WFI, given IV over 30 mins

Infection	Dose (g)	Interval (hr)
Mild–moderate	2	6
Moderate–serious	4	6
Life threatening	4	4

In renal impairment:

CC (ml/min)	Dose (g)	Interval (hr)
10 –20	2 – 4	6 – 12
<10	2 – 4	12

How not to use piperacillin
Not for intrathecal use (encephalopathy)
Do not mix in the same syringe with an aminoglycoside (efficacy of aminoglycoside reduced).

Adverse effects
Hypersensitivity
Haemolytic anaemia
Transient neutropenia and thrombocytopenia
Convulsions (high dose or renal failure)

Cautions
Owing to the sodium content (~2 mmol/g), high doses may lead to hypernatraemia.

TEICOPLANIN

This glycopeptide antibiotic has bactericidal activity against aerobic and anaerobic Gram +ve bacteria.

What to use teicoplanin for
Infections caused by MRSA
Gram +ve endocarditis

How to use teicoplanin
IV: 400 mg stat followed by 200 mg daily
For severe infections: 400 mg 12 hrly for 3 doses, then 400 mg daily
Reconstitute with WFI supplied, given over 3–5 mins

Monitor: FBC
          LFTs

In renal impairment:
Dose reduction not necessary until day 4, then reduce dose as below

CC (ml/min)	Dose reduction	Interval
40 – 60	½	daily
<40	⅓	daily

Adverse effects
Hypersensitivity
Blood disorders
Ototoxic (uncommon)
Nephrotoxic (uncommon)

Cautions
Vancomycin sensitivity
Renal/hepatic impairment
Concurrent use of ototoxic and nephrotoxic drugs

VANCOMYCIN

This glycopeptide antibiotic has bactericidal activity against aerobic and anaerobic Gram +ve bacteria. It is also effective in the treatment of pseudomembranous colitis, for which it is given by mouth. It is not significantly absorbed by mouth. A vancomycin-resistant strain of enterococcus has been seen in Britain.

What to use vancomycin for
Pseudomembranous colitis
Prophylaxis and treatment of endocarditis
Serious infections caused by MRSA

How to use vancomycin
- Pseudomembranous colitis
Orally: 125 mg 6 hrly for 7-10 days
- Endocarditis and MRSA
IV infusion: 500 mg 6 hrly or 1 g 12 hrly, given over at least 60 mins (rate no more than 10 mg/min).
Duration of therapy is determined by severity of infection and clinical response. In staphylococcal endocarditis, treatment >3 weeks is recommended.

Vancomycin must first be reconstituted by adding WFI:
    250 mg vial - add 5 ml WFI
    500 mg vial - add 10 ml WFI
    1 g vial - add 20 ml WFI
The liquid in each reconstituted vial will contain 50 mg/ml vancomycin.

Further dilution is required:
    Reconstituted 250 mg vial - dilute with at least 50 ml diluent
    Reconstituted 500 mg vial - dilute with at least 100 ml diluent
    Reconstituted 1 g vial - dilute with at least 200 ml diluent
Suitable diluent: 0.9% saline or 5% dextrose

Monitor: Renal function
       Serum vancomycin levels (p 9)

How not to use vancomycin
Rapid IV infusion (severe hypotension, thrombophlebitis)
Not for IM administration

Adverse effects

Following IV use:

Severe hypotension

Ototoxic and nephrotoxic

Blood disorders

Hypersensitivity

Rashes

Cautions

Concurrent use of:

aminoglycosides – ↑ ototoxicity and nephrotoxicity

loop diuretics – ↑ ototoxicity

Organ failure

Renal: Reduce dose

ANTI-FUNGAL AGENTS

AMPHOTERICIN B – FUNGIZONE®

Amphotericin B is active against most fungi and yeasts. It is not absorbed from the gut when given orally. When given intravenously it is highly toxic and side-effects are common. The liposomal and colloidal formulations now available are less toxic, particularly in terms of nephrotoxicity.

What to use amphotericin B for

- Intestinal candidiasis
- Urinary candidiasis
- Severe systemic fungal infections:
  Aspergillosis
  Candidiasis
  Coccidiomycosis
  Cryptococcosis
  Histoplasmosis

How to use amphotericin B

- Orally: Intestinal candidiasis
  100-200 mg 6 hrly
- Bladder washout: Urinary candidiasis
  50 mg in 1000 ml 5% dextrose/day per Foley catheter.
- IV: Systemic fungal infections
  250 µg/kg daily, gradually increased if tolerated to 1 mg/kg daily
  For severe infection: 1.5 mg/kg daily or on alternate days
  Available in 20 ml vial containing 50 mg amphotericin
  Reconstitute with 10 ml WFI (5 mg/ml)
  For peripheral administration: Dilute further with 500 ml 5% dextrose (to 0.1 mg/ml)
  Give over 6 hrs

  For central administration: Dilute further with 50-100 ml 5% dextrose
  Give over 6 hrs

Prolonged treatment is usually needed (duration depends on severity and nature of infection).

Monitor: Potassium
             Magnesium
             Creatinine
             FBC
             LFTs

How not to use amphotericin B

Must not be given as IV bolus
Not compatible with saline

Adverse effects

- Fever and rigors
  Common in first week. May need paracetamol, chlorpheni-ramine and hydrocortisone
- Nephrotoxicity
  Major limiting toxicity. Usually reversible
- Hypokalaemia/hypomagnesaemia
  25% will need supplements
- Anaemia (normochromic, normocytic)
  75% . Due to bone marrow suppression
- Cardiotoxicity
  Arrhythmias and hypotension with rapid IV bolus
- Phlebitis - frequent change of injection site
- Pulmonary reactions
- GI upset
  Anorexia, nausea, vomiting

Cautions

Concurrent use of other nephrotoxic drugs and corticosteroids
Hypokalaemia – increases digoxin toxicity.

AMPHOTERICIN B COLLOIDAL DISPERSION – AMPHOCIL®

AMPHOCIL® is a colloidal formulation containing a stable complex of amphotericin B and sodium cholesteryl sulphate. It is available in vials containing either 50 mg or 100 mg of amphotericin B. It is less toxic than the parent compound. Deterioration in renal function attributable to AMPHOCIL® is rare.

What to use colloidal amphotericin B for
Severe systemic fungal infections, when conventional amphotericin B is contraindicated because of toxicity, especially nephrotoxicity.

How to use colloidal amphotericin B
IV infusion: Start at 1 mg/kg once daily, increasing to 3-4 mg/kg once daily, given at a rate of 1-2 mg/kg/hr.

AMPHOCIL® must first be reconstituted by adding WFI:

     50 mg vial – add 10 ml WFI
     100 mg vial – add 20 ml WFI

The liquid in each reconstituted vial will contain 5 mg/ml amphotericin B. This is further diluted to a final concentration of 0.625 mg/ml by diluting 1 volume of the reconstituted amphocil with 7 volumes of 5% dextrose.

Flush an existing intravenous line with 5% dextrose before infusion.

Monitor: Potassium and magnesium
In patients requiring renal dialysis, give AMPHOCIL® at the end of each dialysis.

How not to use colloidal amphotericin B
Must not be given as IV bolus
Not compatible with saline
Do not mix with other drugs

Adverse effects
Prevalence and severity lower than conventional amphotericin B

Cautions
Concurrent use of nephrotoxic drugs and corticosteroids.
Diabetes: AMPHOCIL® contains lactose monohydrate 950 mg/50 mg vial or 1900 mg/100 mg vial. (may cause hyperglycaemia).

AMPHOTERICIN B (LIPOSOMAL) – AmBisome®

A formulation of amphotericin B encapsulated in liposomes. It is less toxic than the parent compound. Each vial contains 50 mg amphotericin. Store vials in fridge 2-8°C

What to use liposomal amphotericin B for
Severe systemic fungal infections, when conventional amphotericin B is contraindicated because of toxicity, especially nephrotoxicity.

How to use liposomal amphotericin B
IV: Initially 1 mg/kg daily, increase gradually if necessary to 3 mg/kg daily

Add 12 ml WFI to each 50 mg vial of liposomal amphotericin B (4 mg/ml)

Shake vigorously for at least 15 s

Calculate the amount of the 4 mg/ml solution required:

i.e.   100 mg = 25 ml
          150 mg = 37.5 ml
          200 mg = 50 ml
          300 mg = 75 ml

Using the 5 micron filter provided add the required volume of the 4 mg/ml solution to at least equal volume of 5% dextrose (final concentration 2 mg/ml) and give over 30–60 mins.

The diluted solution must be used within 6 hrs

How not to use liposomal amphotericin B
Must not be given as IV bolus

Not compatible with saline

Do not mix with other drugs

Adverse effects
Prevalence and severity lower than conventional amphotericin B

Cautions
Concurrent use of nephrotoxic drugs and corticosteroids

FLUCONAZOLE

Antifungal active against candida and cryptococcal infections. It is rapidly and completely absorbed orally. Oral and IV therapy equally effective; IV for patients unable to take orally. Widely distributed in tissues and fluids. Excreted unchanged in urine.

What to use fluconazole for
Local or systemic candidiasis
Cryptococcal infections

How to use fluconazole
- Oropharyngeal candidiasis
  Orally: 50-100 mg daily for 7-14 days
- Oesophageal candidiasis or candiduria
  Orally: 50-100 mg daily for 14-30 days
- Systemic candidiasis or cryptococcal infections
  IV infusion: 400 mg initially, then 200-400 mg daily
  Do not give at rate >200 mg/hr
  Continued according to response (at least 6-8 weeks for cryptococcal meningitis)

How not to use fluconazole
Avoid concurrent use with astemizole or terfenadine (arrhythmias)

Adverse effects
Rash
Pruritus
Nausea, vomiting, diarrhoea
Raised liver enzymes
Hypersensitivity

Cautions
Renal/hepatic impairment
May increase concentrations of cyclosporin, phenytoin (enzyme inhibition)

NYSTATIN

Nystatin is not absorbed when given orally and is too toxic for IV use.

What to use nystatin for
Mucocutaneous and intestinal candidiasis

How to use nystatin
- Oral candidiasis
- 1 ml (100,000 units) 6 hrly, holding in mouth
- Intestinal candidiasis
- Orally: 500,000 units 6 hrly, doubled in severe infections

How not to use nystatin
IV too toxic

Adverse effects
Rash
Oral irritation

ANTI-VIRAL AGENTS

ACICLOVIR

Interferes with herpes virus DNA polymerase, inhibiting viral DNA replication. Aciclovir is renally excreted and has a prolonged half-life in renal impairment.

What to use aciclovir for
- Herpes simplex virus infections
    HSV encephalitis
    HSV genital, labial, perianal and rectal infections
- Varicella zoster virus infections
    Beneficial in the immunocompromised patient when given IV within 72 hrs: prevents complications of pneumonitis, hepatitis or thrombocytopenia.
    In patients with normal immunity, may be considered if the ophthalmic branch of the trigeminal nerve is involved.

What not to use aciclovir for
Not suitable for CMV or EBV infections

How to use aciclovir
IV: 5–10 mg/kg 8 hrly
Available in 250 mg and 500 mg vials for reconstitution
Reconstitute 250 mg vial with 10 ml WFI or 0.9% saline (25 mg/ml), and give over 1 hr.
Alternatively, dilute the reconstituted solution (25 mg/ml) with 0.9% saline to give a concentration not >5 mg/ml, and give over 1 hr.

In renal impairment:

CC (ml/min)	Dose (mg/kg)	Interval (hr)
10 – 20	5	12
<10	2.5	24

How not to use aciclovir
Rapid IV infusion (precipitation of drug in renal tubules leading to renal impairment).

Adverse effects
Phlebitis
Reversible renal failure
Elevated liver function tests
CNS toxicity (tremors, confusion and fits)

Cautions
Concurrent use of methotrexate
Renal impairment (reduce dose)
Dehydration/hypovolaemia (renal impairment caused by precipitation in renal tubules).

GANCICLOVIR

Ganciclovir is related to aciclovir but is more active against cytomegalovirus (CMV). It is also more toxic. It causes profound myelosuppression when given with zidovudine; the two should not be given together particularly during initial ganciclovir therapy.

What to use ganciclovir for
- CMV infections in immunocompromised patients
- Prevention of CMV infection during immunosuppression after organ transplantation

What not to use ganciclovir for
Hypersensitivity to ganciclovir and aciclovir
Abnormally low neutrophil counts

How to use ganciclovir
IV infusion: 5 mg/kg 12 hrly, given over 1 hr through the filter provided.
Reconstitute the 500 mg powder with 10 ml WFI, then dilute with 50–100 ml 0.9% saline or 5% dextrose.
Wear polythene gloves and safety glasses when preparing solution.
Duration of treatment: 7–14 days for prevention and 14–21 days for treatment.
Ensure adequate hydration.
Monitor: FBC
U&Es
LFTs

Adverse effects
Leucopenia
Thrombocytopenia
Anaemia
Fever
Rash
Abnormal LFTs

Cautions
History of cytopenia, low platelet count
Concurrent use of myelosuppressants
Renal impairment

SUGGESTED FURTHER READING

ABPI Data Sheet Compendium
> 1995-96

British National Formulary
> Number 31 (March 1996)

Clinical Anaesthetic Pharmacology
> Edited by JW Dundee, RSJ Clarke and W McCaughey
> Churchil Livingstone 1991

Introduction to Drug Metabolism
> G Gibson and P Skett
> Chapman & Hall 1993

The Pharmacologic Approach to the Critically Ill Patient
> Edited by B Chernow
> Williams & Wilkins 1994

Sedation and Analgesia in the Critically Ill
> Edited by G R Park and R N Sladen
> Blakewell Science 1995

APPENDIX A:

CREATININE CLEARANCE

Severity of renal impairment is expressed in terms of glomerular filtration rate, usually measured by the creatinine clearance. Creatinine clearance may be estimated from the serum creatinine.

Estimating creatinine clearance from serum creatinine:

$$CC \text{ (ml/min)} = \frac{\text{weight (kg)} \times (150 - \text{age})}{\text{serum creatinine (μmol/L)}}$$

In males 10% is added to, and in females 10% is subtracted from the value obtained.

Renal impairment is arbitrarily divided into 3 grades:

Grade	CC (ml/min)
Mild	20–50
Moderate	10–20
Severe	<10

Renal function declines with age; many elderly patients have a glomerular filtration rate below 50 ml/min which, because of reduced muscle mass, may not be indicated by an increased serum creatinine. Similar difficulties may occur with the critically ill, wasted patient. It is wise to assume at least mild renal impairment when prescribing for the elderly.

APPENDIX B:

WEIGHT CONVERSION
(Stones/Pounds to Kilograms)

		Pounds						
		0	2	4	6	8	10	12
Stones	6	38.1	39.0	40.0	40.8	41.7	42.6	43.5
	7	44.5	45.4	46.3	47.2	48.1	49.0	49.9
	8	50.8	51.7	52.6	53.5	54.4	55.3	56.2
	9	57.2	58.1	59.0	59.9	60.8	61.7	62.6
	10	63.5	64.4	65.3	66.2	67.1	68.0	68.9
	11	69.9	70.8	71.7	72.6	73.5	74.4	75.4
	12	76.2	77.1	78.0	78.9	79.8	80.7	81.6
	13	82.6	83.5	84.4	85.3	86.2	87.0	88.0
	14	88.9	89.8	90.7	91.6	92.5	93.4	94.3
	15	95.3	96.2	97.1	98.0	98.9	99.8	100.7
	16	101.6	102.5	103.4	104.3	105.2	106.1	107.0
	17	108.0	108.9	109.8	110.7	111.6	112.5	113.4
	18	114.3	115.2	116.1	117.0	117.9	118.8	119.7

APPENDIX C:

INFUSION RATE

To calculate the infusion rate in ml/hr:

$$\text{Infusion rate (ml/hr)} = \frac{\text{Dose } (\mu g/kg/min) \times \text{Weight (kg)} \times 60}{\text{Concentration of solution } (\mu g/ml)}$$

APPENDIX D:

PAEDIATRIC DRUG DOSES

Adrenaline	10 µg/kg IV (=1 ml/kg of 1:100,000 solution)
Alfentanil	10 µg/kg IV
Amoxycillin	50 mg/kg IV (initial dose in theatre)
Ampicillin	50 mg/kg IV (initial dose in theatre)
Atracurium	0.5 mg/kg IV Increments: 50% loading dose
Atropine	0.02 mg/kg IV/IM; 0.03 mg/kg PO (max 0.5 mg)
Benzylpenicillin	25–50 mg/kg IV (initial dose in theatre)
Calcium chloride (10%)	0.2 ml/kg IV
Cefotaxime	30-60 mg/kg IV (initial dose in theatre)
Codeine	1 mg/kg IM 6 hrly
Diazepam	0.2 mg/kg PO (as premed)
Diclofenac	1 mg/kg PO/PR 8 hrly
Erythromycin	12.5 mg/kg IV over 30 mins
Etomidate	0.3 mg/kg IV
Fentanyl	1 µg/kg IV
Flucloxacillin	25 mg/kg IV
Gentamicin	2.5 mg/kg IV
Glycopyrrolate	0.01 mg/kg IV
Hyoscine	10 µg/kg IM
Ibuprofen	5 mg/kg PO 6 hrly
Ketamine	1-2 mg/kg IV; 5–10 mg/kg IM
Meropenem	10-20 mg/kg 8 hrly IV increasing to 40 mg/kg 8 hrly IV for meningitis.
Methohexitone	1.5-2 mg/kg IV
Metoclopramide	0.15 mg/kg PO/IV/IM 8 hrly
Metronidazole	7.5 mg/kg IV 8 hrly
Midazolam	0.5 mg/kg PO (as premed)

Morphine	0.05–0.2 mg/kg IV; 0.2 mg/kg IM
Naloxone	4 µg/kg IV every 20 mins
Neostigmine	50 µg/kg IV
	For reversal: With atropine 25 µg/kg or glycopyrollate 10 µg/kg. Dilute one ampoule of 2.5 mg neostigmine /0.5 mg glycopyrollate with 0.9% saline up to 10 ml. Give 1 ml for every 5 kg weight.
Pancuronium	0.1 mg/kg IV
	Increments: 20% loading dose
Paracetamol	15 mg/kg PO/PR
Pethidine	1–3 mg/kg IV/IM
Prochlorperazine	0.2 mg/kg IM 8 hrly
Propofol	2–3 mg/kg IV (add lignocaine 1 mg/10 ml propofol)
Suxamethonium	1–2 mg/kg IV
Temazepam	1 mg/kg PO, max 20 mg (as premed)
Thiopentone	Neonates: 2 mg/kg IV Others: 4–6 mg/kg IV
Triclofos	30–50 mg/kg (max 1 g)
Trimeprazine	2–3 mg/kg PO
Vecuronium	0.1 mg/kg IV Increments: 30–50% loading dose

DRUG INDEX